Joint Commission
RESOURCES

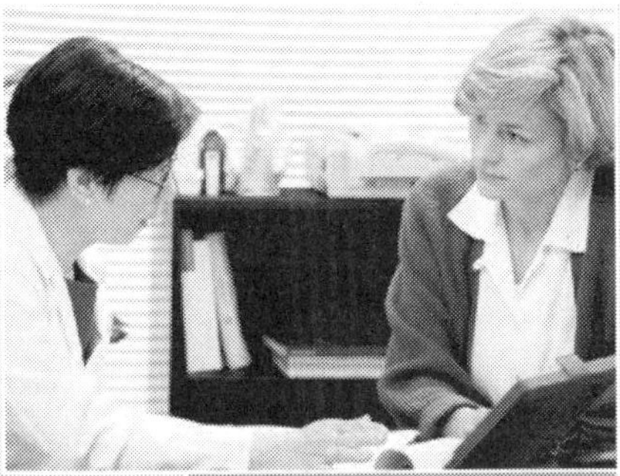

Engaging Physicians in Patient Safety:
A Handbook for Leaders

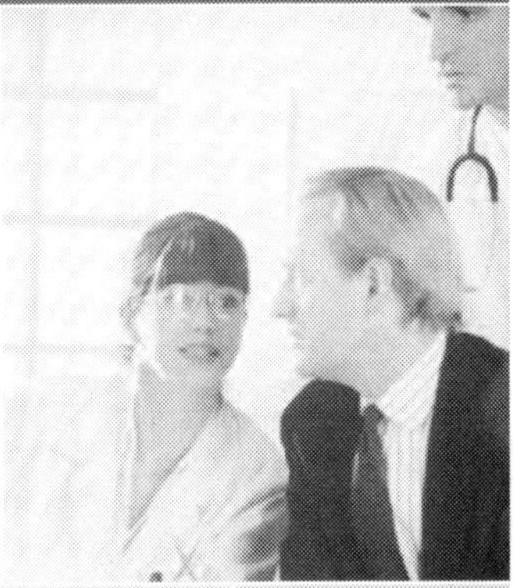

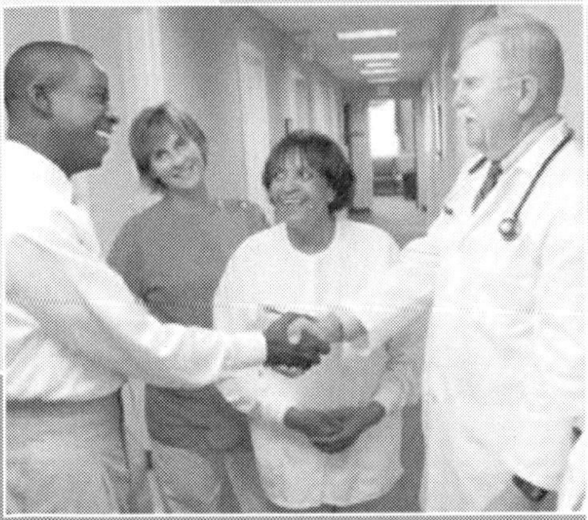

Improving Health Care Quality and Safety

Senior Editor: Ilese J. Smith
Project Manager: Christine Wyllie
Manager, Publications: Eileen Norris
Production Manager: Johanna Harris
Associate Director: Cecily Pew
Executive Director: Catherine Chopp-Hinckley, Ph.D.
Joint Commission/JCR Reviewers: Richard Croteau, M.D.; Darlene A. Christiansen, R.N., L.N.H.A., M.B.A.; Catherine Chopp-Hinckley, Ph.D.; Robert Katzfey

Joint Commission Resources Mission

The mission of Joint Commission Resources is to continuously improve the safety and quality of care in the United States and in the international community through the provision of education and consultation services and international accreditation.

Joint Commission Resources educational programs and publications support, but are separate from, the accreditation activities of the Joint Commission. Attendees at Joint Commission Resources educational programs and purchasers of Joint Commission Resources publications receive no special consideration or treatment in, or confidential information about, the accreditation process.

The inclusion of an organization name, product, or service in a Joint Commission publication should not be construed as an endorsement of such organization, product, or service, nor is failure to include an organization name, product, or service to be construed as disapproval.

Joint Commission Resources, Inc. (JCR), a not-for-profit affiliate of the Joint Commission on Accreditation of Healthcare Organizations (Joint Commission), has been designated by the Joint Commission to publish publications and multimedia products. JCR reproduces and distributes these materials under license from the Joint Commission.

Printed in the U.S.A. 5 4 3 2 1

Requests for permission to make copies of any part of this work should be mailed to:
Permissions Editor
Department of Publications
Joint Commission Resources
One Renaissance Boulevard
Oakbrook Terrace, Illinois 60181
permissions@jcrinc.com

ISBN: 0-86688-946-9
Library of Congress Control Number: 2005928513

For more information about Joint Commission Resources, please visit http://www.jcrinc.com.

Contents

Foreword v

Chapter 1 *An Overview of the Physician's Role in Today's Health Care Safety Environment* 1
- Patient Safety as a Systems Issue 3
- The Status of Patient Safety Efforts 5
- Physician Attitudes Toward Patient Safety 10
- What Hospital Leaders Can Do 16

Chapter 2 *Practical Strategies for Educating Physicians About Patient Safety Initiatives* 23
- Looking at the Current Culture 24
- Building a Culture of Safety 25
- Building a Case for Patient Safety 31
- Planning for Effective Physician Education 34
- Educating Proactively 39

Chapter 3 *Practical Strategies for Involving Physicians in Teams* 47
- Bringing Physicians into the Fold 48
- Enlisting Physician Champions 49
- Setting Up Effective Teams 51
- Developing Team Goals 57
- Providing Training for Performance Improvement Team Members 59
- Allocating Adequate Resources 62

Chapter 4 *Facilitating Physician Participation in Patient Safety* 73
- Defining the Scope of Physician Involvement 75
- Improving Communication 76
- Streamlining Processes 79

Appendix A *Selected Resources* 83

Appendix B *2006 National Patient Safety Goals and the Universal Protocol for Preventing Wrong Site, Wrong Procedure, Wrong Person Surgery™* 91

Index 105

Foreword

Physicians have always been concerned about patient safety. That's one of the main reasons the American College of Surgeons formed the Joint Commission in 1951. Avoidance of medical errors has been an issue for physicians individually, but in today's highly technical health care environment, physicians need to realize that the majority are due to systems failure. The old strategy of finding the physician at fault, taking disciplinary action, demanding retraining, and perhaps setting new policy is not the answer. We must remind ourselves that with all the new diagnostic tools, therapeutic modalities, and procedures, and an aging, sicker population, there are going to be more medical errors. As physicians, we need to be deeply involved in activities to enhance patient safety. This is an excellent opportunity to assume a leadership role as a member of the health care team.

For many years, our professors in medical school led us to believe that physicians were infallible and incapable of making mistakes. That attitude has caused many of our colleagues to be skeptical about medical errors as a reality. This is followed by a lack of motivation to make change or by a concern about loss of autonomy. A final and very real barrier, with increased quotas and financial concerns, is lack of time. One solution to breaking down those barriers is to embrace the team care strategy, working closely with other health care professionals and staff. With the focus on the patient and his/her clinical care, the scope of activity and responsibility can be defined and communication, a critical element, can be improved. A new culture of patient safety can be established.

My experience in encouraging physician engagement in patient safety and quality activities has revealed many positive findings. Physicians are very interested in enhancing patient safety and want to hear about root causes of serious adverse events or solutions (best practices) for patient safety. Each health care organization has a champion or champions of patient safety who provide important motivation to their colleagues. Larger health care systems or community consortia are working together in the interest of patient safety. Many organizations have developed a quality or patient safety council with significant physician membership. These groups meet regularly, with meaningful agendas dealing with improved outcomes, performance measurement, and other issues relevant to physicians. Just as in baseball, physicians need to contribute to the elimination of medical errors and thus achieve the Gold Glove.

William Jacott, M.D.
Special Adviser for Professional Relations
at the Joint Commission

Chapter 1: *An Overview of the Physician's Role in Today's Health Care Safety Environment*

Physicians and hospitals are at a unique juncture in history. Alongside ever-changing advances in medical technology, dwindling staff, and payer insistence on more cost-efficient use of resources, there is a growing demand for evidence of safe, high-quality care and provider accountability for that care.

Numerous government agencies, accrediting organizations, professional societies, employers, insurers, hospitals, and health care professionals are working toward a coordinated effort to measure and improve patient safety. A deliberate overlap in national patient safety expectations allows health care organizations to focus on key initiatives, share and learn from the experiences of other organizations, and use evidence-based practices to build safer processes.

The biggest push for improved safety has occurred in the acute care setting. Of the more than 3,500 sentinel events reported to the Joint Commission between 1995 and the

> Physicians and other hospital leaders must understand that only when human mistakes are accepted as inevitable will it be possible to shift away from a punitive frame of mind and focus on identifying underlying systems failures. The traditional approach of fixing blame, imposing discipline, retraining, and writing new policies will not prevent human error but will stifle discussion and discovery of the causes of error.
>
> —KETRING S.P., WHITE J.P.: DEVELOPING A SYSTEMWIDE APPROACH TO PATIENT SAFETY: THE FIRST YEAR. *JT COMM J QUAL IMPROV* 28:287–295, JUN. 2002.

end of 2005, 87% occurred in a hospital environment; nearly 75% of these events resulted in patient death and an additional 10% in loss of function.[1] Hospitals need all staff to participate in patient safety efforts, if they are to reduce errors and avoid system failures. However, physician participation has often been difficult, if not impossible, to obtain. Considerations such as time constraints, skepticism regarding the need for and usefulness of any interventions, and uncertainty of a team-oriented approach can cause physicians to avoid involvement in improvement activities.

This chapter looks at the importance of patient safety and the present state of initiatives across the country. It also examines some of the reasons for the difficulty in recruiting physicians for these initiatives.

Patient Safety as a Systems Issue

Today's health care system is more complex than ever before, and it is this complexity that has pushed patient safety into the spotlight. An intrinsic need exists to simplify processes and reduce variability in processes so that providers can ensure patient safety. Take, for example, an uncomplicated and routine hernia operation; before the process is completed, the patient will interact with myriad health care professionals in different settings:

- An initial meeting with the primary care physician
- A meeting with a surgeon and an anesthesiologist
- Preoperative laboratory tests and x-rays performed by technicians
- Preoperative care performed by nurses and technicians on the day of surgery
- The surgery itself, involving the surgeon, the anesthesiologist, and other surgical staff
- Postoperative care in the recovery room, including nursing care and examinations by the surgeon and anesthesiologist
- Explanation of discharge instructions by nursing staff

Throughout this entire process, information must move from one person to another and from one site to another. Laboratory work and x-rays have to be ordered, performed, and interpreted correctly, as well as communicated in a timely manner to the surgeon and anesthesiologist. The correct surgical supplies have to be available. Clean, properly maintained equipment needs to be at hand and working properly. Administrative tasks need to be coordinated to facilitate care from different departments, as well as transportation to the operating room and recovery room.[2]

It is difficult to ensure that all the components in this process are completed correctly each time. It is even more difficult after the variables of different physicians, each doing things his or her own way, are introduced. If individual physicians have different processes, operating approaches, recovery procedures, and discharge criteria, it becomes much more difficult to ensure that each step in the process goes as smoothly as it should. Complicating an already complex situation, inexperienced staff, including new residents, may be participating in the process. When processes have many variables, the risk of adverse events increases.

James Reason developed the Swiss Cheese Model as a tool to illustrate the multiple sources of adverse outcomes in complex systems. Figure 1-1 on page 4 shows how this model can work for health care processes and highlights the institutional, organizational, professional, team, individual, and technical layers involved in such processes. Each layer has holes or lapses, and when these holes line up, an error can reach the patient. It is important to note that individuals are only one layer in the model and that most adverse events have more than one

Figure 1-1. *Swiss Cheese Model of Adverse Event Causation*

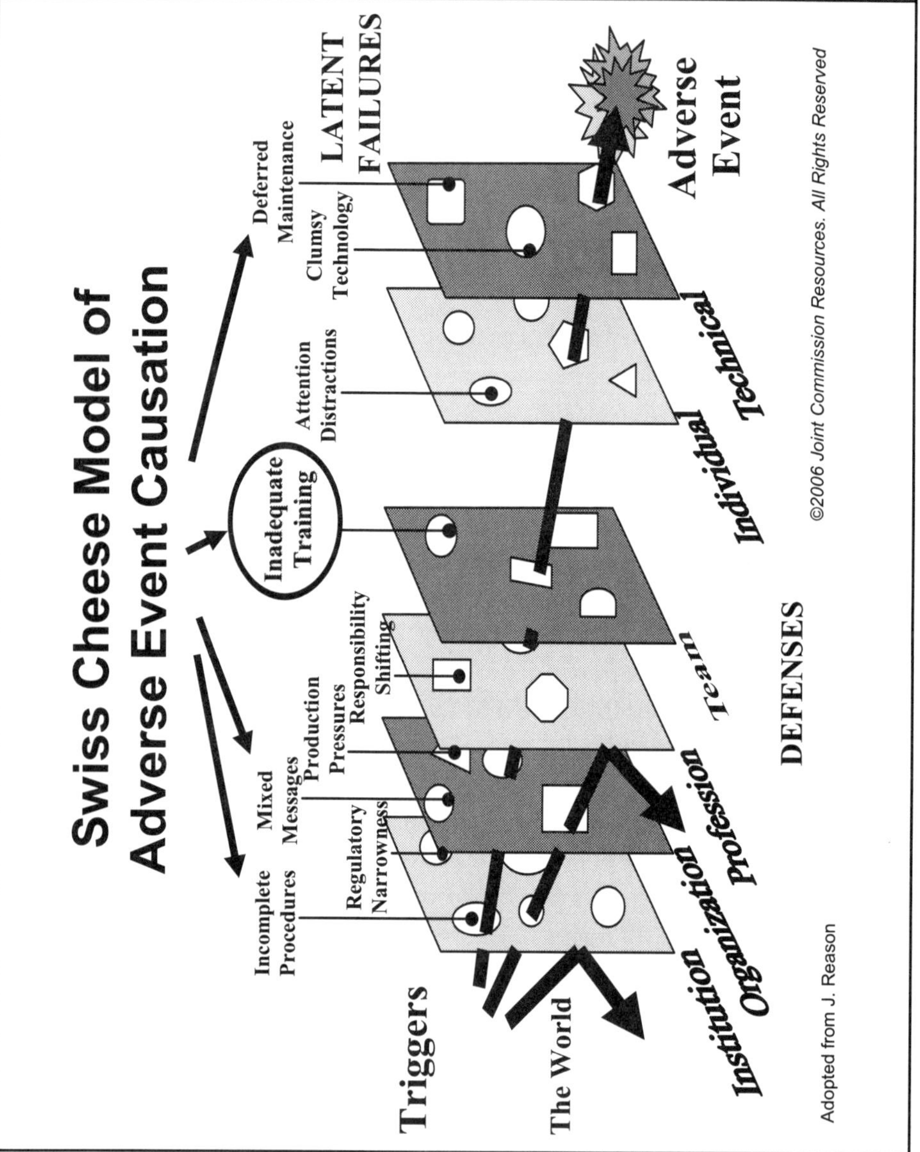

Originally developed by James Reason, this model illustrates how errors can slip through the many layers of a complex process to result in an adverse event.

Source: Angood P.B., Hellman R.: Medical Staff Role in Patient Safety [audioconference]. Oakbrook Terrace, IL: Joint Commission Resources, Inc., 2005.

Table 1-1. *Contributing Factors to Adverse Events*

Cause	Contributing Factors
Individual	Judgment
	Communication
	Teamwork
	Stress
	Compliance with policies
	Fatigue
	Emotions (boredom, frustration)
Environment	Distractions
	Noise
	Ergonomics
	Precautions
	Clutter
	Interruptions
	Lighting
Patient	Behavior
	Language
	Compliance
	Health literacy
	Fear
	Disease acuity

Cause	Contributing Factors
Technology	Design
	Variability
	Availability
	Quality
	Packaging and labeling
	Training
Processes	Staff experience
	Staffing levels
	Supervision
	Competency assessment
	Policies and procedures
	Complexity
	Hand-offs
	Work flow
Leadership	Lack of awareness
	Neglect
	Lack of visibility
	Blame and shame
	Delegation
	Inadequate resources
	Failure to reduce process complexity

Source: *Leadership and Systems Thinking*. Washington, D.C.: National Patient Safety Foundation. http://www.npsf.org (accessed Nov. 21, 2005).

cause. Table 1-1 above lists the numerous factors that can contribute to errors and adverse events. Ensuring safe care is not the sole responsibility of specific caregivers, but an organizationwide effort that involves every function and system in the hospital.

The Status of Patient Safety Efforts

The Institute of Medicine's (IOM's) national reports on patient safety

To Err Is Human: Building a Safer Health System (1999) and *Crossing the Quality Chasm: A New Health System for the 21st Century* (2001) provided additional data on the number of patient deaths that occur each year due to preventable errors, while calling for sweeping changes to measure, improve, and monitor the level of safety in health care organizations. Government agencies, accrediting bodies, third-party payers, and the public began demanding that health care providers be accountable for both safety and patient outcomes. For example, The Leapfrog Group, composed of more than 170 of the largest organizations and companies that buy health care, uses its combined purchasing power to encourage hospitals and physicians to improve the quality and safety of health care. Preference is given to health care providers that implement recommended quality and safety practices, and the group's Web site (http://www.leapfroggroup.org) includes quality ratings for participating hospitals.

The Centers for Medicare & Medicaid Services (CMS) also dedicates part of its Web site to quality-of-care data from participants. *Hospital Compare* (http://www.hospitalcompare.hhs.gov) shows data submitted by more than 4,000 hospitals on 20 measures. These measures reflect recommended treatments for acute myocardial infarction (AMI), heart failure, and pneumonia, as well as the prevention of surgical infections. Sponsored by the Hospital Quality Alliance—a collaborative effort involving CMS, national quality and hospital organizations, accrediting bodies, and others—the Web site updates its results quarterly to allow consumers to learn about the safety and quality of care offered by specific hospitals.

The Joint Commission makes quality data from all surveyed organizations available to the public via the Quality Check page of its Web site at http://www.jointcommission.org. In addition, it has embedded patient safety principles in its standards and releases annual National Patient Safety Goals to promote specific improvements in patient safety (see Appendix B). The goals highlight problematic areas in health care, such as communication, medication use, and patient falls, and describe evidence- and expert-based solutions to these problems (see Sidebar 1-1, page 7). The goals focus on systemwide solutions whenever possible. An outgrowth of the goals is the Joint Commission's Universal Protocol aimed at eliminating wrong-site, wrong-procedure, and wrong-patient surgeries.

Sidebar 1-1. ***Medical Practices Presenting Significant Opportunities for Improving Patient Safety***

Various government agencies, professional associations, and hospital systems continuously work to identify the medical practices that present the greatest risks to patient safety. Only when the problems are known can solutions and best practices be developed. For example, the Agency for Healthcare Research and Quality (AHRQ) published a landmark compendium of literature reviews *Making Health Care Safer: A Critical Analysis of Patient Safety Practice* in July 2001. Based on the expert reviews in this study, AHRQ determined that the following 11 medical practices represent a high level of opportunity for improving patient safety:

- Appropriate use of prophylaxis to prevent thromboembolism in patients at risk
- Use of perioperative beta blockers in appropriate patients to prevent perioperative morbidity and mortality
- Use of maximum sterile barriers while placing central intravenous catheters, to prevent infections
- Appropriate use of antibiotic prophylaxis in surgical patients to prevent postoperative infections
- Asking that patients recall and restate what they have been told during the informed consent process
- Continuous aspiration of subglottic secretions to prevent ventilator-associated pneumonia
- Use of pressure-relieving bedding materials to prevent pressure ulcers
- Use of real-time ultrasound guidance during central line insertion to prevent complications
- Patient self-management for warfarin to achieve appropriate outpatient anticoagulation and prevent complications
- Appropriate provision of nutrition, with a particular emphasis on early enteral nutrition in critically ill and surgical patients
- Use of antibiotic-impregnated central venous catheters to prevent catheter-related infections

According to AHRQ, focusing analysis and improvement efforts on these high-priority areas can help organizations more safely deliver care.

Source: Landry M.D., Sibbald W.J.: Changing physician behavior: A review of patient safety in critical care medicine. *J Crit Care* 17:138–145, Feb. 2002.

Professional associations, national health care organizations, and hospitals are also joining the push for a safer health care experience. The American Medical Association (AMA) has launched a Making Strides in Safety campaign to educate physicians on ways to enhance patient safety in hospitals. AMA President John C. Nelson, M.D., M.P.H., noted that the campaign draws much-needed attention to the patient safety movement and provides physicians and other health care professionals with specific strategies to meet an attainable goal: "The AMA's position has always been [that] one preventable error is one too many. This campaign will allow the AMA to help physicians help their patients while improving health care safety."[3]

The Institute for Healthcare Improvement (IHI) has launched the 100,000 Lives campaign, through which it will work with other organizations to disseminate improvement tools and supporting expertise throughout the U.S. health care system. The goal of this national patient safety initiative is to save 100,000 lives by June 2006 by accelerating the pace of improvement in U.S. hospital care through consistently implementing proven life-saving interventions. Numerous groups—including the AHRQ, American College of Physicians, AMA, CMS, Joint Commission, National Association for Healthcare Quality, National Patient Safety Foundation, and Veterans Health Administration—are participating in the campaign.

The initial IHI interventions include the following:

- Deploying rapid response teams where staff at any level can call on a specialty team to examine a patient at the first sign of decline. (The team responds to the patient's needs in minutes rather than hours.)
- Delivering reliable, evidence-based care for AMI to prevent deaths from heart attacks, including beta blockers and aspirin at admission; ACE inhibitors, reperfusion, and beta blockers at discharge; and smoking-cessation counseling as appropriate.
- Preventing adverse drug events by implementing medication reconciliation practices—a formal process of identifying the most accurate list of all medications a patient is taking; comparing them against physicians' admission, transfer, and/or discharge orders; notifying the physician of discrepancies; and documenting needed changes.
- Preventing central line infections by implementing a series of

interdependent, scientifically grounded processes, including hand hygiene, barrier precautions, chlorhexidine skin antisepsis, catheter site and administration protocols, and no routine catheter replacement so as to discontinue use as quickly as possible.

- Preventing surgical-site infections by reducing risk factors and optimizing evidence-based processes of care, including antibiotic prophylaxis guidelines, appropriate hair removal, and perioperative glucose control.
- Preventing ventilator-associated pneumonia by implementing a series of interdependent, scientifically grounded processes, including elevating the head of the bed by 30 degrees, peptic ulcer prophylaxis, deep venous thrombosis prophylaxis, intermittent lightening of sedative use, and strict hand-washing norms.

Hospitals participating in this campaign are required to submit two sets of data: profile information, including number of licensed beds, teaching status, average daily census, and so on; and monthly acute care inpatient mortality data (the number of inpatient deaths and discharges for a given calendar month, excluding stillborn, emergency department (ED)–only, and observation patients who are generally not considered admitted or discharged). Hospitals can also submit data for intervention-level measures, such as codes per 1,000 discharges (a rapid response team intervention-level measure) and percentage of AMI patients receiving aspirin at arrival (an AMI care intervention-level measure). Hospitals can use these data to measure the progress of their work at a more detailed level.[4] As of June 2005, more than 2,200 U.S. acute care hospitals had joined the campaign.

With all this attention, it would seem that the field as a whole has accepted the importance of improving patient safety and is working toward improvements. Unfortunately, this is not the case. According to Lucian L. Leape, M.D., most hospitals do not have active safety programs, and only a handful of hospitals have made significant progress toward creating nonpunitive environments that will encourage incident reporting and better patient safety. He cites three major barriers to improving patient safety: lack of national leadership, lack of commitment by hospital leaders, and lack of physician involvement and leadership: "Most of the leaders of the patient safety movement are, in

> One of the major lessons that health care has had to learn from other safety-conscious industries is that the pervasive medical culture of individual responsibility and blame stands in the way of efforts to make health care safer. No amount of individual reprimand will change the fact that all providers will err from time to time. The goal is thus to develop a system that recognizes, and even expects, these occasional human failures and minimizes the chance they will result in patient harm.
>
> —Shojania K.G., Wald H., Gross R.: Understanding medical error and improving patient safety in the inpatient setting. *Med Clin N Am* 86:847–867, 2002.

fact, physicians. But the majority of physicians are not on board; they are watching from the sidelines. They are too busy and are not convinced there is a problem."[5]

Why is it so difficult to convince physicians to participate in patient safety initiatives? After all, in looking at the more than 3,500 sentinel events that were reported to the Joint Commission between 1995 and 2005, it is plain that the majority of root causes associated with these events are systems issues that somehow affect or are affected by physicians (Figure 1-2, facing page). Does a simple lack of time and knowledge of the data explain physicians' reluctance, or are other factors at work?

Physician Attitudes Toward Patient Safety

It is impossible to identify one particular reason that physicians are often not involved in patient safety improvement programs; a combination of many factors is most likely responsible. As with anyone else, physicians' willingness to take on perceived extra responsibilities depends a great deal on how they feel about other aspects of their work. Some elements of physician satisfaction include quality of care, level of autonomy, compensation, relationships with patients and colleagues, and the practice environment.[6] Specific demographic characteristics, including age, gender, and geographic area, have also been found to

Figure 1-2. *Root Causes of Sentinel Events*

Total Number of Sentinel Events Reviewed by the Joint Commission Since January 1995	3,548

Type of Sentinel Event	#	%
Patient suicide	464	13.1%
Wrong-site surgery	455	12.8%
Op/postop complication	444	12.5%
Medication error	358	10.1%
Delay in treatment	269	7.6%
Patient fall	189	5.3%
Patient death/injury in restraints	138	3.9%
Assault/rape/homicide	121	3.4%
Perinatal death/loss of function	109	3.1%
Transfusion error	94	2.6%
Infection-related event	67	1.9%
Patient elopement	66	1.9%
Fire	65	1.8%
Anesthesia-related event	58	1.6%
Medical equipment–related	56	1.6%
Maternal death	51	1.4%
Ventilator death/injury	43	1.2%
Infant abduction/wrong family	23	0.6%
Utility systems–related event	19	0.5%
Unintended retention of foreign body	13	0.4%
Other less frequent types	446	12.6%

All 12 of the most commonly identified root causes of sentinel events involve physicians in some way, even if only peripherally. Communication, compliance with specific procedures, care planning, and organizational culture are some of the areas in which physicians' cooperation (or lack of it) can significantly impact patient safety.

Source: Joint Commission on Accreditation of Healthcare Organizations: Root Causes of Sentinel Events, http://www.jointcommission.org.

affect satisfaction. For example, dissatisfaction tends to be higher among physicians who are younger, female, practicing in urban settings, putting in long hours, and dealing with compromises in quality of care.[6]

Training and academic background also contribute to physicians' perceptions of their work. Medical school prepares them to work well with physiological systems rather than organization- or people-oriented systems. Physicians have been taught to focus on their individual patients, and many see patient safety efforts that improve conditions for populations as interfering with that focus. Because criticism among medical colleagues is generally frowned upon, physicians tend to be uncomfortable discussing adverse events among themselves. This discomfort leads to missed opportunities for learning from each others' experiences and providing support.[7] Physicians also face the ever-present fear of litigation, which builds resistance to having performance measured and to making quality and safety data accessible to others.

Physicians must consider their own interests as well as those of their patients, hospitals, society, and third-party payers. Throw in concerns about professionalism and competence, and an unwillingness to admit to a lack of knowledge or request help,[8] and it is easy to see how complex their motivations are. All these motivations, characteristics, and background considerations likely form the basis for the four major barriers to physician participation in patient safety efforts: skepticism, the fear of losing autonomy, time constraints, and a lack of motivation to change.

Skepticism

This barrier has two distinct elements: skepticism about the need for patient safety interventions, and skepticism about the efficacy of those interventions. Most physicians believe that the IOM's estimate of 98,000 preventable deaths per year is exaggerated, and because some errors are inevitable, they are basically unmanageable. These physicians feel that the costs of health care, malpractice insurance, and lawsuits are far more important.[9] Because errors are a natural part of the process, it follows that incident reporting and attempts to eliminate errors are pointless.[10]

Part of the problem may be the perception that data relating to safety and clinical practice are inadequate and/or unreliable. Often, hospital leaders, risk managers, and performance improvement staff present generalized data for specific populations in ways that the majority of physicians cannot easily understand. Clinicians are naturally suspicious of data that are confusing (whether because of the lack of specificity or the uncontrolled variables) and question whether these data are actually comparable to their own patients' situations.[11]

Even when physicians are convinced that a problem with patient safety exists, they may not believe that measurement and improvement activities will help. As noted by one doctor of science and his coworkers, most physicians believe that individuals are more likely to be responsible for medical errors than systems are.[9] Other researchers reported similar findings; physicians are more likely to talk to patients about cost of treatment than about safety or quality of care, believing that only the high quality of their own skills prevents their patients from being harmed.[12] Performance improvement is viewed as a waste of time. There may be several reasons for this type of skepticism, including lack of knowledge regarding evidence that supports interventions, a perception of limitations to existing evidence, and/or a belief that effective interventions cannot be adapted and properly implemented in one's hospital.[13] Whatever the reason, a lack of physician support makes it far more difficult (if not impossible) to realize improvements in patient safety.

Autonomy

With the ever-growing complexity of care, physicians must rely on any number of organizational supports—including multidisciplinary care teams, computer-aided decision support systems, electronic medical records, and well-designed care processes—to provide safe, high-quality care.[14] However, autonomy in practice and the right to lead are important to all physicians. Medical schools train physicians to make difficult clinical decisions on their own rather than to work as part of a team. The level of discretion clinicians have about the way they practice, including the availability of specific medications and utilization of diagnostic procedures, greatly influences their overall job satisfaction.[15] Many physicians see patient safety interventions, clinical practice guidelines, and performance improvement activities as threats to their autonomy.

Clinicians also tend to have a healthy distrust of administrative personnel and other nonphysicians, who they believe may use safety or improvement data as an excuse to exert more control over medical decisions. Interestingly, although younger physicians and residents are more willing to collaborate within a team framework,[16] the degree of distrust they feel toward organizations and hospital leaders is even higher than that of more experienced physicians.[11] Such feelings may certainly contribute to the skepticism exhibited toward both patient safety data and the efficacy of interventions discussed earlier.

Time Constraints

A 2003 study of family practitioners, general internists, pediatricians, general surgeons, and obstetrician-gynecologists (ob-gyns) reported the following results for a 12-year period[17]:

- Physician work hours remained stable or decreased slightly.
- Annual and hourly incomes increased significantly for family practitioners, general internists, and pediatricians, and negligibly for general surgeons; incomes for ob-gyns decreased.
- There was no evidence that time spent in direct patient care activities decreased.

Despite these findings, many physicians feel that they need to work harder and see more patients to maintain their incomes. Whether because of capitation or limitations imposed by third-party payers or hospitals, clinicians' perceptions are that they spend less time with their patients and may not always be able to provide the diagnostics, treatment, and/or medications they deem necessary.

Financial cutbacks to reduce hospital expenses can, indeed, impose clinician time constraints. Physicians may find themselves with more responsibility for paperwork because fewer secretaries are available. Also, limited staffing means that nurses (many of them part-time or contract staff) are not as familiar with inpatients' situations and make more frequent phone calls to physicians; the information nurses provide during these calls may be incomplete or inappropriate because they do not understand what physicians need to know. As a result, orders are delayed and the level of clinician frustration increases.[11]

Physicians are needed as leaders in patient safety efforts, but leadership takes time—from organizing and participating on teams, to reviewing baseline and benchmark data, to developing and/or revising processes, to serving as advocates and opinion leaders among medical staff. Given the perception that regular patient care and administrative duties take up more time than ever, it is not surprising that physicians are reluctant to commit extra effort to uncompensated activities that can seem overwhelming. That's especially true when they often deem such activities as unnecessary and ineffectual.

Lack of Motivation

Physicians receive few, if any, rewards for improving patient safety. Payment systems are generally the same no matter what the quality of care or outcomes achieved. Many states do not require reports on errors that result in patient death or serious harm.[14] A study conducted by the National Patient Safety Foundation found that physicians view the current culture as having the following characteristics[18]:

- Tolerance (it is permissible to commit errors)
- Denial (both health care organizations and physicians refuse to see a problem)
- Complacency (some errors are considered preventable, while others are considered business as usual)
- Hierarchical (it is unlikely that patients or other health care professionals would speak up if they thought something was wrong)

> Changing individual behavior requires motivators and the "unfreezing" of individuals' preference for the status quo. In terms of structural change, an organization must change its focus from its existence or costs to outcomes.
>
> —Cohen M.M., Eustis M.A., Gribbins R.E.: Changing the culture of patient safety: Leadership's role in health care quality improvement. *Jt Comm J Qual Safe* 29:329–335, Jul. 2003.

Physicians also identified the historically punitive reaction to adverse events as a barrier to incident reporting. The combination of these factors makes it more likely that an adverse event will occur and less likely that it will be reported or analyzed.

With no motivation to change, physicians cling to habit and continue to use familiar processes, regardless of recommendations to the contrary.

What Hospital Leaders Can Do

It is clear that although the four basic barriers to physician participation in patient safety are distinct, they are also completely interdependent. Each compounds and strengthens the others to the point that hospital leaders may begin to see physicians as more problematic than the safety risks they are trying to address. This book provides ways to deal with the barriers already discussed, at the same time considering their interdependence and the prevailing physician mind-set.

Because change can never occur until clinicians see the need and possibility for it, Chapter 2 focuses on building a learning culture in which incident reporting, open discussion of errors and near misses, and multidisciplinary collaboration are commonplace. This type of culture sets the stage for educating physicians about problems in patient safety, regulatory and other requirements, how improved safety affects their patients, and how patient safety activities can become part of the hospital routine. Chapter 3 examines ways to build multidisciplinary teams that include physicians and characteristics of successful teams. The problem of time constraints is addressed in Chapter 4, which provides techniques hospital leaders can use to streamline both day-to-day routine and patient safety activities to use physicians' time most effectively. Appendix A contains a list of resources, including journal articles and Web sites that may be helpful to those working to bring physicians into the patient safety fold. Finally, Appendix B contains a list of the 2006 National Patient Safety Goals for hospitals and the Universal Protocol for Preventing Wrong Site, Wrong Procedure, Wrong Person Surgery™.

Change can only occur when everyone in an organization—leaders, physicians, clinical staff, and support staff—makes a commitment to work together to make it happen. *Engaging Physicians in Patient Safety: A Handbook for Leaders* is a tool to help hospital leaders achieve that commitment to better patient safety.

CASE STUDY
University of Michigan Health System

The University of Michigan Health System (UMHS) in Ann Arbor, Michigan, has joined eight other Michigan health care systems (see Sidebar 1-2, page 18) in an effort to improve patient safety. Launched in April 2005, Hospitalists as Emerging Leaders in Patient Safety (HELPS) is targeting the following patient safety initiatives:

- Developing techniques for performing quality improvement research so physicians can accurately assess the effects of their efforts in clinical and patient care
- Preventing device-related infections
- Eliminating medication errors and creating a culture of safety
- Improving the use of preventive medications for surgical patients
- Closing gaps in care between different hospital services and those that occur when patients are discharged from the hospital
- Improving intensive care practices, including pneumonia prevention
- Improving end-of-life care, including pain management and formulating advance directives
- Increasing safety for older patients, including fall risk reduction and preventing delirium through cognitive stimulation activities for patients who experience delirium
- Learning lessons from patient safety efforts[19]

Participating organizations have agreed to focus on these nine initiatives as well as their own hospital-specific initiatives. The main initiatives were selected based on HELPS organizations' needs, patient safety data, and national patient safety initiatives.

Funded by a $117,000 grant from the Blue Cross Blue Shield of Michigan Foundation, HELPS team members consist of hospitalists, patient safety leaders, and quality improvement leaders from each of the participating organizations. HELPS has intentionally targeted hospitalists to develop systems-based solutions. According to Scott Flanders, M.D., chief of hospitalist services at UMHS, "Unlike doctors in private practice, who have to juggle caring for their patients both in and out of the hospital, hospitalists can focus entirely on managing the complex needs of patients while they're in the hospital.

Sidebar 1-2. ***Participating HELPS Health Systems***

The combined patient discharges for these health care systems total 80,000 each year.

- Beaumont Hospital
- Chelsea Community Hospital
- Detroit Medical Center
- Henry Ford Health System
- St. John Health System
- Oakwood Healthcare System
- St. Joseph Mercy Healthcare System
- University of Michigan Health System
- VA Ann Arbor Healthcare System

"Working with hospitalists facilitates patient safety initiatives. By changing the practice patterns of a smaller number of physicians (hospitalists), you can have a positive effect on a large number of patients. General medicine is difficult to target; hospitalists allow this to happen. We want to do with general medical care what specialists have done in the past. Hospitalists also know their institutions the best and how to get buy in from other physicians."

The HELPS agenda has been planned for the next two years so that each of the nine patient safety initiatives will be addressed at a face-to-face meeting of the nine member organizations. These evening meetings are planned four to six times each year and will be scheduled two to three months in advance to allow members to juggle their schedules and ensure attendance. If the primary representative from a hospital or system is unable to attend, he or she will send a designee. Representatives will present on their organizations' experiences for their selected patient safety initiative.

To maximize the effectiveness of meeting times, the structure of the presentations has also been established:

- A review of the literature about best practices
- A presentation of analyzed data collected from all participating institutions, as well as any available national data against which to benchmark performance
- Feedback from members about attempted interventions
- Identification of factors that led to success or failure in the presenting organization's efforts
- Identification of barriers
- Discussion of methods to facilitate change related to patient safety and quality improvement

The regular meetings give representatives a chance to share tips, tools, and techniques. These representatives will then take the information back to their individual organizations to implement within their existing performance improvement systems.

Between meetings, the group will perform site visits at member organizations to troubleshoot, look for opportunities to improve patient safety, and provide assistance on specific patient safety projects that are in progress. HELPS plans to maintain communication and provide support via a listserv. The group is also creating a Web-based survey to solicit feedback from members on the overall project to see what could be improved.

References

1. *Sentinel Event Statistics.* Oakbrook Terrace, IL: Joint Commission on Accreditation of Healthcare Organizations, Dec. 31, 2004. http://www.jointcommission.org (accessed Oct. 19, 2005).
2. Lawrence D.: *From Chaos to Care: The Promise of Team-Based Medicine.* Cambridge, MA: Perseus Publishing, 2002, pp. 114–116.
3. AMA joins campaign to save 100,000 lives [press release]. Chicago: American Medical Association, Dec. 15, 2004.
4. *How-To Guide: Submitting Data for the 100,000 Lives Campaign.* Cambridge, MA: Institute for Healthcare Improvement, 2004.
5. Buerhaus P.I.: Lucian Leape on patient safety in U.S. hospitals. *J Nurs Scholarsh* 36:366, Winter 2004.
6. Haas J.S.: Physician discontent: A barometer of change and need for intervention. *J Gen Intern Med* 16:496–497, Jul. 2001.
7. Aasland O.G., Forde R.: Impact of feeling responsible for adverse events on doctors' personal and professional lives: The importance of being open to criticism from colleagues. *Qual Saf Health Care* 14:13–17, 2005.
8. Smith W.: Evidence for the effectiveness of techniques to change physician behavior. *Chest* 118:8S–17S, Feb. 2000.
9. Blendon R.J., et al.: Views of practicing physicians and the public on medical errors. *N Engl J Med* 347:1933–1940, 2002.
10. Waring, J.J.: Beyond blame: Cultural barriers to medical incident reporting. *Soc Sci Med* 60:1927–1935, 2005.
11. Weinberg R.M., Bhatt N.V., Vogenberg F.R.: Engaging physicians in cost savings initiatives: Eliminating medication cost bias in the selection of inpatient medications. *Physician Exec* pp. 12–18, Jan./Feb. 2005.
12. Goode L.D., et al.: When is "good enough"? The role and responsibility of physicians to improve patient safety. *Acad Med* 77:947–952, Oct. 2002.
13. Rosen A.B., et al.: Physicians' views of interventions to reduce medical errors: Does evidence of effectiveness matter? *Acad Med* 80:189–192, Feb. 2005.
14. Richardson W.C., Corrigan J.M.: Provider responsibility and system redesign: Two sides of the same coin. *Health Aff* 22:116–118, Feb. 2003.
15. Ramirez A.J., Graham J.: Mental health of hospital consultants: The effects of stress and satisfaction at work. *Lancet* 347:724, 1996.
16. Sorokin R., Riggio J.M., Hwang C.: Attitudes about patient safety: A survey of physicians-in-training. *Am J Med Qual* 20:70–77, Feb. 2005.
17. Weeks W.B., Wallace A.E.: Time and money: A retrospective evaluation of the inputs, outputs, efficiency, and incomes of physicians. *Arch Intern Med* 163:944–948, 2003.
18. VanGeest J.B., Cummins D.S.: *An Educational Needs Assessment for Improving Patient Safety: Results of a National Study of Physicians and Nurses* [white paper]. National Patient Safety Foundation, 2003. http://www.npsf.org/download/EdNeedsAssess (accessed Oct. 19, 2005).

19. Teaming up for patient safety: Hospital-based doctors across SE Michigan launch program to protect patients from errors [press release]. University of Michigan Health System, Apr. 13, 2005.

Chapter 2: *Practical Strategies for Educating Physicians About Patient Safety Initiatives*

Education about the value of patient safety initiatives is the first step in changing the existing mindsets of physicians. Clinicians need to understand why such initiatives are necessary, what can be accomplished, and how patient care can be improved. They also need to believe that patient safety is a top priority for the hospital and that leaders and staff are willing to put in the time, effort, and money required to make care safer.

Education is most effective when it takes place in an organizational environment that fosters learning and the free exchange of information, without fear of reprisals or blame. Companies in the manufacturing industry work to build cultures of safety that provide this type of environment and encourage employees at all levels from all departments to bring up problems they observe, as well as suggestions for solving those problems. Cultures of safety are just as (if not more) important in hospitals, where the

> You can't just "change the culture"—you have to link this to solving a real problem.
>
> —Paul G. Preston, M.D., anesthesiologist, assistant chief of quality, Kaiser Permanente Medical Center, San Francisco. In Critical Events Team Training, presented at *Moving from the Sidelines to the Frontlines of Patient Safety: Empowering the Medical Staff*, Joint Commission Resources, Inc., Chicago, Sep. 29–30, 2005.

report of a near miss can lead to a proactive effort to change a process and prevent future risks to patients.

Looking at the Current Culture

According to a 2003 National Patient Safety Foundation (NPSF) study,[1] most physicians view the current hospital culture as having the following characteristics:

- Tolerance of errors
- Denial of problems (by both organizations and clinicians)
- Complacency (by which some errors are considered serious and others are business as usual)
- Hierarchical (making it unlikely that patients or other staff will speak up if they think something is wrong)

The combination of these cultural characteristics makes it more likely that adverse events and near misses will occur, and less likely that they will be reported or analyzed. Because unreported incidents can never be used as educational opportunities to prevent future adverse events, the likelihood of true improvement is reduced and the current culture is perpetuated.

The first three characteristics were discussed in Chapter 1, but hierarchy deserves a special mention here because it interferes with properly coordinated care and inhibits staff from speaking up about safety concerns. Hierarchy creates additional patient safety risks and works against a culture of safety; when staff members do speak about problems to physicians or leaders, the conversation tends to be indirect and/or deferential. New and inexperienced staff may hold back information or concerns, for fear of repercussions or due to insecurity about their roles in the hospital or on a team. And senior staff members may resist feedback from someone they view as a subordinate.[2] Although the full effect of hierarchy's negative impact on communication may be difficult to quantify, it can act as a significant barrier to patient safety in many situations, including between surgical team members in the operating room, care delivery team members in the emergency room, and physicians and nurses during the hospital discharge process.

One of the best examples of hierarchy interfering with safety-related communication may be the situation faced in teaching hospitals. Residents, who are often the first to respond to adverse events and may observe issues that are overlooked by more experienced staff, are reluctant to share their observations with their attending physicians.[3] Clinicians in training feel that they must prove themselves to the physicians who are evaluating them, and that to admit to a mistake or a near miss may negatively affect the level of confidence and trust they are trying to establish.

Fear of repercussions is not limited to residents. In the NPSF study, only 50% of physicians surveyed believed that they worked in a non-punitive environment. The perception that mistakes will automatically result in blame prevents many health care professionals from taking part in patient safety initiatives, reporting actual or potential errors, and admitting to mistakes. Before a culture of safety can be achieved, any lingering "bad apple" perceptions must be dispelled.

Building a Culture of Safety

Hospital leaders are continually challenged to address the concerns of both internal and external stakeholders while delivering the highest-quality, safest care possible. How they respond to these challenges and the example they set for clinical and support staff plays a key role in how successful their organizations will be. Sidebar 2-1, page 26, lists some of the behaviors required of leaders to demonstrate their commitment to change and to encourage others in the hospital to do the same.

According to Peter M. Senge, director of the Systems Thinking and Organizational Learning Program at the Massachusetts Institute of Technology, Sloan School of Management, leaders need to concentrate on building learning organizations in which all daily activities are viewed as opportunities to learn and expand knowledge. He summarizes leaders' essential role as follows[4]:

> In a learning organization, leaders' roles differ dramatically from that of the charismatic decision maker. Leaders are designers, teachers, and stewards. These roles require new skills: the ability to build shared vision, to bring to the surface and challenge prevailing mental models, and to foster more systemic patterns of thinking. In short, leaders in learning organizations are responsible for building organizations where people are continually expanding their capabilities to shape their future—that is, leaders are responsible for learning.

This shift away from traditional management philosophies is also evident in the concept of principle-centered leadership promoted by Stephen R. Covey, founder and chairman of the Covey Leadership Center and the Institute for Principle-Centered Leadership in Provo, Utah. This concept focuses on a humanistic approach to leadership, and how leaders interact with and understand other people at all levels and in all areas of their organizations. Some of the key traits Covey lists as characteristic of principle-centered leaders include service oriented, continually learning, and synergistic.[5] The last is important because it means they are able to build cohesive, successful teams and negotiate win-win solutions to problems. They also exercise a belief in other people, which helps create a climate for growth and eliminate workers' fear of participation in projects.

Sidebar 2-1. ***Leadership Behaviors to Encourage Physician and Staff Commitment to Change***

- Identify and communicate a vision and values.
- Integrate desired changes into all hospital systems (for example, through recognition and reward).
- Keep physicians and staff informed on topics related to the "big picture" for the hospital.
- Treat physicians and staff as assets and ask for input.
- Role model any new behaviors expected of physicians and staff.

Source: Phillips, K.M.: *The Power of Health Care Teams: Strategies for Success*. Oakbrook Terrace, IL: Joint Commission on Accreditation of Healthcare Organizations, 1997, p. 25.

Addressing patient safety effectively means taking a proactive approach—looking for glitches in the system

> Implementation of redesigned care processes is always a difficult task for health care delivery organizations. Key to successful implementation is strong clinical leadership throughout project conception, design, implementation, and evaluation. Physicians will need to lead this effort, will need to be educated in these approaches, and will need to be assured that implementation will not lead to loss of control of their patients or loss of revenue.
>
> —Classen D.C., et al.: The roles and responsibility of physicians to improve patient safety within health care delivery systems. *Acad Med* 77:963–972, Oct. 2002.

before they result in adverse events. Leaders who are committed to learning understand that ignoring problems does not make them go away, it just lets them continue until they cause even bigger problems. These leaders believe in taking a proactive systems approach and focus on questions such as "What could go wrong with this process?" or "How can we fix this process before (more) negative outcomes occur?" rather than "Whose fault is this?" This attitude helps steer away from the traditional culture of attributing blame for mistakes.

Leaders and staff in learning organizations look at adverse events and near misses from the perspective that these situations are variations in a process or system. (Remember the Swiss Cheese Model from Figure 1-1 on page 4.) They analyze systems to determine how and why events have occurred, or might occur in the future, rather than focusing on who made a mistake. For example, most learning organizations have moved away from the traditional morbidity and mortality conferences, which tended to look for individuals who were responsible for errors, and toward meetings in which multidisciplinary teams perform root cause analyses. Physicians play a critical role in this process, bringing clinical expertise and experience to error analysis and systems planning/redesign.

Learning organizations also recognize the value of near misses.

Events that do not result in adverse patient outcomes but have the potential to do so can provide a powerful learning opportunity for health care professionals. The aviation industry has demonstrated that less severe mistakes and near misses present the chance to analyze systems in a psychologically safer, lower-risk situation with less possibility for group tension, disagreement, or defensiveness. Instead, assumptions about work processes can be challenged and debated freely among all staff.[6] This allows for practical safeguards to be built into processes to reduce the probability of an adverse event and provide an early warning system to ensure that errors are identified before they reach the patient.

The Agency for Healthcare Research and Quality (AHRQ) has developed a Hospital Survey on Patient Safety Culture to help organizations assess their patient safety culture. Sections on the participant's primary work area/department, his or her direct supervisor, and the hospital as a whole address issues such as interdepartmental cooperation and respect, effective communication, error reporting and feedback, and overall patient safety rating. The survey also includes recommendations and guidance on sampling, setting up the survey for Web-based completion, and analyzing the data. It is available free of charge on the AHRQ Web site http://www.ahrq.gov/qual/hospculture.

Hoff and coworkers studied the individual and group "best practices" associated with a learning culture and found similarities in areas such as systems thinking, empathy toward others, reciprocal communication, and collaborative inquiry.[6] The checklist in Sidebar 2-2, page 33, adapted in part from the results of that study, may provide a starting point for a questionnaire for soliciting feedback from clinical staff and other employees to help leaders determine how far their hospitals have progressed toward becoming learning organizations with cultures of safety.

Considerations in the Academic Environment

It would seem that the easiest place to build a learning environment would be in teaching hospitals; however, leaders of these organizations may find it just as difficult to encourage error reporting and open discussion of safety issues as do their counterparts in nonacademic settings. Several authors agree that the best time to teach physicians to be collaborative and bring them into the patient safety/quality improvement fold is when they are still in training.[3,7–9] As mentioned earlier, residents may be afraid to admit to mistakes or point out errors on the part of others, for fear of appearing incompetent or antagonizing supervisors. If attending physicians are uncomfortable with reporting and collaboration, they may also make clinicians in training more reluctant to participate.

Linda A. Headrick, M.D., Ph.D., Professor of Medicine at Metrohealth Medical Center, Case Western University, has described a conceptual model she and colleagues have found effective in helping students, teachers, and others see the value of educating new clinicians with an eye to improving care quality.[9] Known as the Education Compass, this model allows providers and learners to see the benefits and costs of quality improvement for all the stakeholders involved. To use the compass, each of the points illustrated in Figure 2-1, page 30, are examined from the viewpoint of clinicians, patients, the hospital, and any other important stakeholders. The compass points are interpreted as follows:

- *Clinical:* specific, formal assessments of the results of clinical care and education
- *Functional:* how well people or organizations representing different perspectives (such as patients, hospitals, teachers, residents, the community) can do what they need to do when clinical care and education are present
- *Satisfaction:* how those representing different perspectives react to the processes of clinical care and education
- *Cost:* the resources expended by each of the different perspectives for clinical care and education

Education is at the center of the compass and influences all points.

The compass can be applied to any process that has been identified as needing improvement or that may pose risks to patient safety. Say that an academic hospital wishes to proactively work on its medication process to reduce the risk of adverse drug events. To show all clinical and support staff how education and improvement in this area will benefit them and other stakeholders, leaders can go through the Education Compass with representatives from each group. For example, all stakeholders would probably identify the important outcome at the clinical point of the compass as excellent patient outcomes with no

Figure 2-1. *The Education Compass*

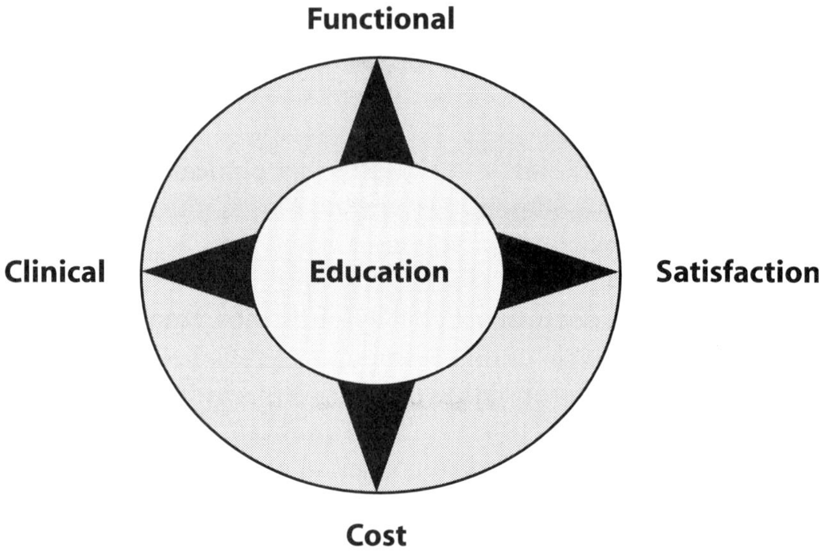

Each of the points of the compass can be applied to the various stakeholders of a process to determine the benefits and costs of improvement and give providers and learners a view of the "big picture."

Source: Ogrinc G.S., et al.: Understanding the value added to clinical care by educational activities. *Acad Med* 74(10):1080–1086, Fig. 2, 1084, Oct. 1999. Used with permission.

adverse drug events. Patients may see the desired outcome for the functional point as effective pain management and a high level of function; clinicians may say that processes such as prescribing and verifying verbal orders are carried out efficiently and effectively. The cost outcome for the patient may be the reduction of out-of-pocket expenses by using the appropriate medications, thus avoiding dangerous drug interactions and reducing the need for additional treatment. For physicians and residents, the outcome may be cost-effective use of formulary drugs to help contain expenditures and allow for safe, high-quality care and high-quality education. This model can be used by any hospital to illustrate what effects improving safety through education can have.

Building a Case for Patient Safety

> ... if you incorporate physician leadership development and support as a part of your organizational change effort, you're more likely to be successful and gain the benefit of building capabilities to support the next initiative. Strong, capable physician leadership with appropriate organizational structures to support them may be all you need for successful change initiatives, either large or small scale.
>
> —Mark B. Wenneker, M.D., consulting manager, The Bard Group. In *Bringing Doctors on Board: Cultivating Physician Leaders and Reducing Pushback*. Manasquan, NJ: The Healthcare Intelligence Network, 2005.

After leaders have committed to a learning environment and a culture of safety and begun to work on making it a reality, they have a basis for educating physicians about patient safety. Perhaps the most difficult goal is to gain clinicians' interest and belief in the importance of safety initiatives and their effects on the clinicians' practice. Physician leadership plays a key role in getting other clinicians to support improvement efforts. Leaders such as the chief medical officer (CMO) can help shape a hospital's safety and improvement goals, as well as balance administration's views of cost–benefit trade-offs. Several authors agree that, when physicians are involved in governance and system design, communication among medical staff, managers, and boards improves; trust is also built with clinical staff by assuring them that their views and goals are represented.[10–12] For example, the chief executive officer of Missouri Baptist Medical Center in St. Louis forged a symbolic and operational partnership with the hospital's CMO that set the tone for and encouraged greater collaboration between hospital managers and physician leaders.[11] The Health Alliance of Central New York, based in Syracuse, New York, redesigned its entire performance improvement system to create shared governance and accountability (and mutual incentives) among administrative and medical leaders.[12] The importance of physician opinion leaders and champions is discussed in more detail later in this chapter and in Chapter 3.

The next challenge is persuading physicians to believe that change is necessary. Most professionals in any field believe that "if it's not broken, don't fix it." It is much easier to maintain the status quo than to expend time and energy on change that might not even be helpful. Some clinicians see the push for improvement in patient safety as nothing but the latest trend in the ever-changing health care field. They must be shown why change is necessary. One way to do this is to present a well-thought-out case for change that looks at where the hospital is now, where it needs to be and why, and how it can get there. Key questions to answer include the following[13]:

- What problems exist in the current environment and what effect do they have?
- What will happen if no change occurs?
- Why should action be taken now?
- How will success be measured? How will things be different?
- What will change require?
- What is the cost of changing versus the cost of staying the same?

Sidebar 2-2, page 33, illustrates how these questions might be used to build a case for improving the ordering process to prevent medication errors. Leaders should try to be as specific, honest, and complete as possible when answering these questions and developing a case. The results can form the basis for team goals in patient safety projects (see Chapter 3).

The Question of Benefits

When trying to engage physicians in patient safety, one of the most important questions leaders will answer is what benefits clinicians will realize from change. Although obviously concerned with their patients' well-being and care, they also want to know how patient safety improvements will make the care process more efficient from their point of view. It is often helpful to focus on technological solutions to problems physicians have identified in a risk-prone process. For example, the hospital in Sidebar 2-3, pages 34–35, might decide to establish a computerized physician order entry (CPOE) system to help eliminate handwriting and transcription errors. Using a CPOE can also help clinicians ensure that dosage, form, and frequency are appropriate, and that potential drug interactions are avoided.

Sidebar 2-2. *Is Your Hospital a Learning Organization?*

Use the following questions as a starting point to solicit opinions from physicians, clinical staff, and other employees about your hospital's culture.

	Yes	No
Are you encouraged to report adverse events and near misses on an ongoing basis?		
Have you been trained in how to make a report?		
Is the reporting process easy to use? For example, are forms readily available, do you know to whom reports should be forwarded, and so on?		
Do you feel comfortable reporting errors without fear of repercussions?		
Do you feel comfortable talking with medical and hospital leaders about patient safety issues and experiences?		
Are reports used to proactively address process improvements?		
Have you participated in system analysis/root cause analysis based on error reports?		
If so, were you encouraged to voice your opinions and participate in discussions?		
Do you receive feedback on reported errors and near misses?		
If you see a threat to patient safety within your area of the hospital, do you feel comfortable speaking up at the time?		
If you see a threat to patient safety in another area of the hospital, do you feel comfortable speaking up at the time?		
Do you feel comfortable talking with other staff members in your area about patient safety issues and experiences?		
Do leaders set shared goals for the hospital that place a high priority on patient safety?		
Do leaders have regular contact with staff, including physicians, nurses, and other clinical staff?		
Do leaders promote interdepartmental and multidisciplinary collaboration throughout the hospital?		
Are leaders willing to explore nontraditional solutions to identified process problems?		
Have you participated in team projects or initiatives to improve patient safety?		
If so, were you given sufficient time to participate and also perform your regular duties?		
Were you given sufficient resources to accomplish the team's stated goals?		
Do you feel that clinical/patient care needs are treated with equal importance to administrative/financial needs?		
Have you observed problems with communication between different areas/departments in the hospital?		
If so, have you reported these problems?		

Of course, the efficacy of CPOEs and various computer-based decision support systems available to support physicians depends entirely on the willingness and ability of those physicians to use them. Convincing clinicians of the importance of making changes to promote safety is only part of the equation; leaders need to provide education to make participation possible.

Planning for Effective Physician Education

A key component of physician participation in patient safety is education: information about existing statistics, risk management, and the need for change; training in skills such as collaboration and

Sidebar 2-3. *Making a Case for Improving the Prescribing Process*

Scenario

Leaders at the fictitious Good Care Hospital have noted a 25% increase in the number of medication errors reported by the quality improvement department during the past 12 months. After performing a root cause analysis, they find that approximately 50% (13) of the errors were related to the ordering process—such as illegible handwriting and misunderstood verbal orders. Only two of the errors reached the patient and no serious harm occurred.

The leaders propose to work with physicians, nurses, and pharmacists to revise the process to eliminate future errors.

Why Change Needs to Occur and What Will Happen If It Doesn't

Although double-checks are in place, the fact that two errors got through to patients means there is a risk that more incidents could occur and result in adverse reactions, serious harm, or death. The ordering process needs to be revised to reduce this risk.

If changes are not made, patients may suffer adverse reactions, serious harm, or death, and legal proceedings may be taken against the hospital and the physician(s) involved.

What Action Needs to Be Taken Now

The pharmacy and therapeutics committee, chief medical officer, nurse manager, director of pharmacy, and office manager will suggest members to be included in a multidisciplinary team to examine the ordering process, identify weaknesses, and develop solutions. The team will report directly to the CEO and quality management committee. A time line for completion of the project will be set within two weeks of the first meeting.

continued on next page

performance improvement techniques that help physicians participate effectively in team activities; and education in new processes to improve safety. Getting the message through to clinicians has proved difficult for most hospitals, whether due to a lack of willingness on the receiving end or incorrect techniques on the transmitting end.

According to the NPSF study mentioned earlier, more than 80% of physicians surveyed recognized that patient safety is an important issue, and nearly 84% recognized the need for physician education and training in patient safety.[1] Respondents identified the following areas as those in which they would like to receive additional education:

Sidebar 2-3. *Making a Case for Improving the Prescribing Process*

continued from previous page

How the Situation Will Change and How Success Will Be Measured

The goal of the project is to make the ordering process more efficient and less prone to error. This should ultimately mean less time spent by physicians, nurses, and pharmacists in questioning and verifying orders; fewer delays in medications reaching patients should also be noted. Care will be safer for patients.

Success will be measured through the existing data collection and analysis process performed by the quality management department. Medication error data will be broken out by type of error, with monthly reporting on order-related errors. Results should show at least 50% improvement in 6 months and 95% improvement in 12 months.

What Will Be Required to Make Changes

- To study the process, identify problems, and develop solutions, time must be allotted for team members to participate in the project.
- Resources needed for a new process will depend on the solutions suggested by the team, but time and money for education must be allotted. All staff and clinicians who participate in the ordering process will need time for education, and more time may be needed for writing, taking, and verifying orders until a "learning curve" has been passed.
- Data collection and analysis are already being performed; extra breakdown can be handled by updating software fields.

The Cost of Change Versus the Cost of Maintaining the Status Quo

- Process changes will cost physician/staff time and budgetary allowances.
- Keeping an error-prone process may cost patient lives or injury, as well as millions of dollars in damages and legal fees.

- Health care error and patient safety definitions
- Technology and patient safety
- Human factors affecting patient safety
- Physician communication
- Systems-level error reporting and analysis
- Error and injury disclosure to patients and their families
- Systems thinking and cultural change
- Nonpunitive environments and systems for reporting errors
- Safety practices
- Models for error reduction

Hospital leaders are responsible for planning and implementing education throughout their organizations. Given that some physicians are already motivated to learn more about the various aspects of patient safety, it is to the leaders' advantage to discover what those aspects are and to work with them accordingly. Planning and implementing include allocating adequate resources to provide effective education, and this has been a sticking point for many hospitals. Although they provide a great deal of educational material, physicians don't seem to take away an understanding of or belief in the topic. Just as medications must be delivered by appropriate routes, patient safety education must be delivered by appropriate methods to engage physician interest and understanding.

Reports in the literature have found that traditional attempts to educate physicians and change behavior have centered around passive methods such as lectures and distributing printed materials.[14–16] Although these methods are time- and cost-efficient in the short term, they have generally proved ineffective (meaning education needs to be repeated and costs more in the long term). As a result, more interactive strategies such as the following are gaining acceptance:

- *Academic detailing.* Also referred to as "one-on-one education"[16] or "educational outreach,"[17] this is a process in which clinical educators interact with individual physicians and staff members to promote desirable medical practices for improved outcomes. For example, the West Virginia University Pharmacy School and the state's Public Employees Insurance Agency have instituted a program in which registered pharmacists visit physicians on site to provide evidence-based information on how various pharmaceuticals can be used effectively for various diseases. The program is aimed at achieving positive patient outcomes while containing medication costs for patients and payers.[17]

Academic detailing has been ranked as one of the most effective education techniques. The best results have been achieved when process-oriented measures rather than outcomes are used.

- *Audit and feedback.* In this process, individual physician usage data are collected and reviewed. Physicians receive the data as feedback about their care processes and patient outcomes, and their numbers can be compared to national or hospital benchmarks or evidence-based standards. Opinions on the efficacy of this method are split: Some sources found that it had minimal effect, some saw moderate results, and others recognized significant change.
- *Simulation of preferred practices.* This strategy offers many advantages to improving patient safety, with no actual risk to patients. Simulations can be performed in workshops addressing practices such as effective communication or by using technology such as computer-based programs and mannequins. Educators can present numerous scenarios and use real medical equipment with the mannequins. Simulations also allow educators to see how team members interact and to determine where team training may be needed.[18]
- *Reminder systems.* With this strategy, physicians can be prompted to follow specific care guidelines via computerized prompts in patient records or other applications such as CPOE systems. Such prompts are based on evidence-based practice and not the individual physician's own patient data. This strategy has proved moderately effective.
- *Debriefings.* These focused meetings can address issues at any level of complexity and include critical incident debriefing, intake rounds and morning reports, and in-services/workshops to address key tasks and skills such as computer use and documentation.[2]
- *Local opinion leaders.* Respected physicians assume leadership roles in championing best practices within a specific region or

> "The presence of a "culture of safety" is particularly important since even the best physicians or providers have a less-than-complete scope of awareness of the potential effects of their interventions."
>
> —Richard Hellman, M.D., F.A.C.E., F.A.C.P., chair, Patient Safety Committee and vice president, American Association of Clinical Endocrinologists; co-chair, Implementation Committee, Physicians Consortium for Performance Improvement. In Improving patient safety in diabetes care in hospital settings—a team effort. Presented at *Moving from the Sidelines to the Frontlines of Patient Safety: Empowering the Medical Staff*, Joint Commission Resources, Inc., Chicago, Sep. 29–30, 2005.

system. Several studies found that this strategy has a positive effect on changing physician behavior. Similar to the academic detailing strategy, its success may be due to the direct interaction physicians have with peers and other health care professionals.

Because most of these education methods are more time intensive than traditional methods, many physicians and hospitals rely on Internet sites for education. From the physician's point of view, Web-based learning has several advantages[20]: easy accessibility, privacy, a choice in level of detail, and timeliness. However, clinicians are most likely to use the Internet when seeking information about a specific patient problem rather than as a learning tool for safety-related topics such as infection control or patient assessment. Although 209 continuing medical education (CME) sites existed in 2001, only 17% of those sites were interactive and 7% were based on recognized clinical practice guidelines.[20] Text-only sites tend to have the same level of effectiveness as other passive forms of education such as seminars and (electronic or hard copy) material distribution; thus, hospitals that plan to use Web- or intranet-based learning tools need to supplement those tools with more interactive strategies. For example, a recent study aimed at designing a Web site to educate physicians about the need for specific disease screening combined such features as needs assessment and tailored learning modules, an interactive response format, and evidence-based content with audit and feedback to increase retention.[20]

Patient Safety Resources

Hospitals need to assume responsibility for educating physicians about national patient safety information, such as the causes of adverse events and ways to prevent them, as well as organization-specific patient safety initiatives. Educators can find a large volume of free material online from government, professional, academic, and other groups. Table 2-1 on pages 40–41 lists some of the resources available, including links to sites that offer CME credit in safety-related areas (additional resources are listed at the end of this book). Because many Web sites offer a huge amount of information on a variety of safety topics, it may be helpful to limit the suggested reading for physicians to pages that relate to areas of specific concern to the hospital. Printing out copies or e-mailing Web links to individual pages will have more impact if physicians can use the information in their daily activities and in association with hospital safety initiatives.

Educating Proactively

Decisions about what method(s) to use for education will be influenced by what topics are to be taught. For example, opinion leaders may be best for getting initial buy-in from physicians, whereas a combination of reminder systems and audit and feedback may work best to change behaviors within a process. Hospital leaders must look at their organization's specific needs and allocate education resources accordingly. When assessing those needs, it is important to remember that some education should take place before the relevant skills are actually required. For instance, because most physicians are used to working and making decisions on their own, they need training in collaborative skills such as active listening to help them work on patient safety teams. Chapter 3 talks more about setting up effective teams and ensuring clinician participation.

Table 2-1. *Online Patient Safety Education Resources*

Agency For Healthcare Research and Quality http://www.webmm.ahrq.gov	Features expert analysis of adverse events reported anonymously in multiple specialties. Access to cases requires online registration. CME credits are offered for completion of Spotlight modules only.
American College of Physicians http://www.acponline.org/ptsafety/index.html	Offers a set of seven modules addressing systems (such as changing culture), medication errors, office design for outpatient care, electronics (such as automated medical records), communication, the role of patients in patient safety, and human cognition.
Joint Commission International Center for Patient Safety http://www.jcipatientsafety.org	This site is designed to serve as a major central repository of resources and information related to all aspects of patient safety that will be relevant for patients, families, physicians, nurses, and pharmacists, as well as for all health care institutions and allied professionals. Provides patient safety products and services (audio conferences, publications, education programs, e-learning courses) and complimentary patient safety resources and tools (case studies, good practice examples, awards, and links to other patient safety resources).
Medscape from WebMD http://www.medscape.com	Provides continuing education activities by specialty for physicians and other health care professionals. Registration is required for CME.

continued on next page

Table 2-1. ***Online Patient Safety Education Resources*** **continued**

continued from previous page

National Patient Safety Foundation http://www.npsf.org	The NPSF has partnered with the Medical College of Wisconsin to offer physicians CME credits (category 1) for a set of 12 modules that address topics such as systems thinking, using technology, team communication, physician-patient communication, learning from mistakes, disclosing injuries and errors, retrospective analysis, and technologies for error reduction.
Society of Academic Emergency Medicine http://www.saem.org/download/patsfty.pdf	Offers a series of seven modules that address awareness of error, definitions and models of error, cognitive error and medical decision making, learning from others' experience, complications from invasive procedures, medical error from a systems perspective, and living with the reality of error.
VA National Center for Patient Safety http://www.va.gov/ncps/index.html	Offers a patient safety tool kit with curriculum, slide presentations, handouts, and assessments. Also includes alerts and newsletters.

CASE STUDY
Brooke Army Medical Center

Organizations can use any number of education methods to get patient safety information to physicians. For example, Brooke Army Medical Center (BAMC) in San Antonio, Texas, created a video-based distance-learning program to disseminate the Joint Commission's National Patient Safety Goals to all staff, including physicians, and discuss how to use the goals to help prevent medical errors and promote patient safety.

A 220-bed health care facility, BAMC is a center for graduate medical education, houses the Institute of Surgical Research, and is certified as a Level 1 trauma center. Medical center staff oversees the Great Plains Health Care Support area, which encompasses 14 states and 8 medical treatment facilities. In addition, BAMC supports the health care services provided to a beneficiary population of more than 573,000 active duty soldiers, their family members, and retired service members and their families in the 14-state support area.

Getting the Information Out

In 2003, the dietetic internship director, who was also a member of BAMC's patient safety and performance improvement functional management team, headed the development of a distance-learning program that would distribute information about the Joint Commission's current goals as well as other performance improvement information to the staff at the eight health care organizations within its support area. Because adult learners usually want specific just-in-time information that is relevant to their immediate problems or concerns, the project team of patient safety experts and media specialists wanted something that would be succinct, easily accessible, and memorable to get across the necessary information. They decided to create a series of two- to three-minute videos that staff could access via an intranet site. Each goal was split into three video segments (*or motion picture expert groups* [MPEGs]), which covered the following:

- Sentinel events that had been reported pertaining to that goal
- Root causes and risk-reduction strategies
- Army Medical Department and BAMC follow-up recommendations and policies

In addition, the team developed MPEGs addressing the FOCUS-PDCA methodology and the importance of effective communication between patients and providers.

Putting It Together

The distance-learning program took 14 months to complete and included the following steps:

- Writing the scripts
- Narrating the scripts on video and adding graphics
- Editing the tapes
- Compressing the videos into a Web-based video format
- Linking the videos to the hospital's intranet site
- Writing the endorsements that were sent out with each video

The scripts for the videos were based on information from leaders in patient safety and clinical care, including the U.S. Pharmacopeia's Center for the Advancement of Patient Safety, American Association for Respiratory Care, American Academy of Orthopaedic Surgeons, Institute for Safe Medication Practices Prevention Emergency Care Research Institute, and U.S. Department of Defense (DoD) Patient Safety Center. BAMC's patient safety and quality services staff helped edit the scripts and approved them before production.

The Fort Sam Houston Army installation, where BAMC is located, has its own television studio; and media specialists from this division were responsible for shooting, producing, and editing the video segments. The tapes were compressed into a digital video format that could be sent as e-mail attachments and placed on the hospital's intranet. The final 34 segments were linked to a special icon on all user desktops, so staff could view the videos simply by clicking on the icon.

The video links were e-mailed on a weekly basis to more than 3,000 BAMC staff members during a six-month period. To emphasize the importance of the information to all disciplines, an endorsement and photograph of a key hospital leader (physician, nurse, administrator, or educator) was e-mailed along with each module or batch of segments. The new video links were posted on the intranet after the e-mails were sent to the BAMC staff members.

Hospital staff members could watch them in groups or alone, on the intranet site or as part of the weekly e-mails. To meet mandatory patient safety training requirements, BAMC required that participation in the distance-learning program be addressed in competency evaluations for all staff. Although participation was not mandatory, the hospital leaders encouraged staff members to look at the videos and sign off on their patient safety training.

Benefits of the Program

By using the digital video format for education, BAMC was able to provide cost-effective, standardized, systematic training that was easily accessible to all hospital staff. Continuous reinforcement was achieved through the ongoing release of modules, each of which contained short, succinct presentations of information. The buy-in and support of senior leaders from all areas helped show staff members that patient safety was a priority for their organization.

The modules were so popular that they were put into use by the DoD and all branches of the military. The videos themselves can be accessed on the DoD, Medical Command, and Army Knowledge Management Web sites as well.[21]

References

1. VanGeest J.B., Cummins D.S.: *An Educational Needs Assessment for Improving Patient Safety: Results of a National Study of Physicians and Nurses* (white paper). National Patient Safety Foundation, 2003. http://www.npsf.org/download/EdNeedsAssess (accessed Nov. 25, 2005).

2. National Patient Safety Foundation: *Leadership and Systems Thinking.* Washington, D.C.: National Patient Safety Foundation. http://npsf.org (accessed Oct. 25, 2005).

3. Sorokin R., Riggio J.M., Hwang C.: Attitudes about patient safety: A survey of physicians-in-training. *Am J Med Qual* 20:70–77, 2005.

4. Senge P.: The leader's new work: Building learning organizations. *Sloan Management Review* pp. 7–23, Fall 1990.

5. Covey S.: *Principle-Centered Leadership.* New York: Summit Books, 1991, pp. 33–39.

6. Hoff T.J., Pohl H., Bartfield J. Implementing safety cultures in medicine: What we learn by watching physicians. *Advances in Patient Safety: From Research to Implementation* (Volume I). Rockville, MD: Agency for Healthcare Research and Quality, pp.15–38.

7. Rosen A.B., et al.: Physicians' views of interventions to reduce medical errors: Does evidence of effectiveness matter? *Acad Med* 80:189–192, Feb. 2005.

8. Goode L.D., et al.: When is "good enough"? The role and responsibility of physicians to improve patients' safety. *Acad Med* 77:947–952, Oct. 2002.

9. Headrick L.A.: The Education Compass: Providing a new direction for education and quality care improvement. *Joint Comm Benchmark* 1:8–9, Jun. 2000.

10. Lambert M.J.: The chief medical officer's evolving role. *Healthcare Exec* 62–63 May/Jun. 2005.

11. Cohen M.M., Eustis M.A., Gribbins R.E.: Changing the culture of patient safety: Leadership's role in health care quality improvement. *Jt Comm J Qual Saf* 29:329–335, Jul. 2003.

12. Hosler F.W., Nadle P.A.: Physician-hospital partnerships: Incentive alignment through shared governance within a performance improvement structure. *Jt Comm J Qual Improv* 26:59–73, Feb. 2000.

13. Palmer B.: *Making Change Work: Practical Tools for Overcoming Human Resistance to Change.* Milwaukee: ASQ Quality Press, 2004, p. 25.

14. Trowbridge R., Weingarten S.: Educational techniques used in changing provider behavior. In Shojania K.G., et al. (eds.): *Making Health Care Safer: A Critical Analysis of Patient Safety Practices.* Evidence Report/Technology Assessment No. 43 (prepared by the University of California at San Francisco– Stanford Evidence-based Practice Center under Contract No. 290-97-0013), AHRQ Publication No. 01-E058. Rockville, MD: Agency for Healthcare Research and Quality, 2001, pp. 601–606.

15. Smith W.R.: Evidence for the effectiveness of techniques to change physician behavior. *Chest* 118(2 suppl):8S–17S, 2000.

16. Landry M.D., Sibbald W.J.: Changing physician behavior: A review of patient safety in critical care medicine. *J Crit Care* 17:138–145, Feb. 2002.

17. Kasprak J.: *West Virginia's Prescription Drug Academic Detailing Program.* Release No. 2005-R-0050. Jan. 5, 2005. http://www.cga.ct.gov/2005/rpt/2005-R-0050.htm (accessed Nov. 25, 2005).

18. Gaba D.M.: Anesthesiology as a model for patient safety in health care. *BMJ* 320:785–788, 2000.

19. Weinberg R.M., Bhatt N.V., Vogenberg F.R.: Engaging physicians in cost savings initiatives: Eliminating medication cost bias in the selection of inpatient medications. *Physician Exec* pp. 12–18, Jan./Feb. 2005.

20. Casebeer L.L., et al.: Designing tailored Web-based instruction to improve practicing physicians' preventive practices. *J Med Internet Res* 5(3):e20, 2003. http://www.jmir.org/2003/3/e20 (accessed Nov. 25, 2005).

21. Jaghab D., et al.: Using a distance-learning program to educate staff on the Joint Commission National Patient Safety Goals. *Jt Comm J Qual and Safe* 30:671–675, Dec. 2004.

Chapter 3: *Practical Strategies for Involving Physicians in Teams*

Just as care delivery does not occur in isolation, no one group or department alone can improve the safety and quality of care. The diversity of patients, the increase in chronic illnesses, and the growing complexity of care delivery are overwhelming for any individual to manage. Physicians need to be part of a multidisciplinary team that brings together the right mixture of necessary skills and experience to create meaningful change. Teamwork is important not only in complex and dynamic environments, such as operating rooms and emergency departments, but also in hospitalwide patient care and improvement processes.

Effective teams do not happen by accident. Team members must learn to communicate with each other, work together, and make decisions together outside the traditional confines of their training and experience. Building a team mentality among clinical staff takes time, patience, and support.

> Your strongest tool [to gain physician buy-in] is making the physicians feel like owners. Give them responsibility and a role in decision making, and you'll have them on board.
>
> —Manuel Lowenhaupt, M.D., national practice leader, CapGemini. In *Recommended Methods for Incenting Doctors*. Healthcare Intelligence Network, Sep. 27, 2005. Available at http://www.hin.com.

Leaders must be willing to back teams in every respect, including the following:

- Creating an infrastructure that sustains teamwork
- Assigning the right people to the right teams
- Setting goals and limitations for teams
- Allocating adequate resources to allow teams to meet their goals
- Providing adequate training for team members

The creation of a learning environment in which physicians and staff work together toward improving patient safety was discussed in Chapter 2. This chapter deals specifically with leaders' responsibilities regarding clinician participation in teams.

Bringing Physicians into the Fold

When physicians consider being part of a team, most of the barriers already discussed in Chapter 1 come to the forefront: skepticism about the need for or usefulness of a team, lack of motivation, the need and desire for autonomy, and time constraints. Leaders must use a variety of methods to overcome these barriers. Many of these methods echo those used to gain clinician buy-in to the importance of patient safety as a whole.

Physicians must be able to see the advantages to working within a team structure. How will their participation benefit them and their patients? Here are some points to bring up in discussions[1–3]:

- *Patient focus.* Emphasizing the patient as the ultimate winner in any safety effort is a good beginning. The main objective of any improvement project is to make care better and safer for the patient, which is also the physician's primary goal.

- *Medical staff input.* Processes cannot be designed or redesigned well without the help of those involved. Clinicians may often complain that processes are not tailored to their needs, but those needs cannot be understood or taken into account unless members of the medical staff contribute their experience and knowledge to (re)design efforts. Physician participation also ensures that teams focus on processes that are most relevant and of greatest concern to the medical staff.
- *Better working conditions.* Clinicians need to see that investing a certain amount of time in building effective communication and working with other health care professionals in a team format can pay off in processes that run more smoothly, require less effort, and generally save them time and frustration. Successes that have been realized in other areas of improvement can be used as examples of the practical usefulness of teamwork.
- *Business aspects.* Although many physicians have their own private practices, outcomes that affect the hospital(s) at which they are privileged affect them as well. In addition to reducing risks to patients, patient safety efforts can eventually decrease overall hospital costs by making processes more efficient. Documented evidence of improved patient safety can be used as a marketing tool to make a hospital more competitive within its geographic area, and can lead to national recognition for both the organization and its staff. None of these benefits can be realized without multidisciplinary teamwork.

Because many physicians may view with skepticism the administrative assurances about the value of teams, the most effective strategy for obtaining buy-in may be to enlist the help of physician champions (also called *early adopters* and *opinion leaders*).

Enlisting Physician Champions

Physicians are most likely to be receptive to team participation when another physician advocates such participation. Therefore, it is important to find clinicians who recognize and speak out for an initiative's

> Improvement in health care delivery . . . is almost always an interdisciplinary process, requiring the expertise and collaboration of everyone who works in the system to be redesigned. The professionals involved must be ready to contribute their own knowledge and skills and be willing to learn from the expertise of others. Each must also be aware of differences such as language and methods of work that, unrecognized, can interfere with effective collaboration.
>
> —Aron D.C., Headrick L.A.: Educating physicians prepared to improve care and safety is no accident: It requires a systematic approach. *Qual Saf Health Care* 11:168–173, 2002.

purpose and scope. Given the opportunity and the necessary tools, these clinicians can build consensus among their colleagues.

Leaders need to identify and cultivate physician champions within their hospital. Champions are not necessarily current medical staff leaders; they may come from the front line, representing the physicians and staff who will be affected by process changes and improvements. The search for champions should be held in all areas affected by a planned patient safety initiative to ensure that an effective support system for change is in place. For example, the champion for a team that is trying to improve rates of hepatitis B virus (HBV) vaccination in newborns may be a hospitalist on the maternity/neonatal floor. This clinician may have one-on-one meetings with the chief of the hospital medical staff and other physicians to help gain support. He or she may note important statistics (90% of perinatal HBV infections can be prevented by administering the HBV vaccine within 12 hours of birth[4]); acknowledge barriers such as inconvenience and a possible lack of reimbursement by insurers; and discuss the errors (incorrect laboratory results, poor communication, and so on) that might lead to a high-risk infant not being vaccinated. This information can have much more impact when delivered by a fellow physician, and paves the way for others to participate in and advocate redesigning processes to ensure that vaccinations are performed.

Physician champions who are committed to safety and a learning culture can also help break down barriers based on hierarchy. As noted in Chapter 2, junior physicians and other caregivers may feel uncomfortable pointing out potential problems, mistakes, or near misses to physicians and senior leaders. This reluctance to speak up can also inhibit staff contributions in team meetings; the fear of possible reprisal, ridicule, or simply being ignored may keep front-line staff and others from expressing valuable ideas and insights. A physician champion who models respect for other team members and openness to their opinions makes a valuable contribution to the team and the overall hospital culture. Champions can ease the way to building collaboration among disciplines and making everyone feel more at ease. For example, a champion may introduce herself using her first name ("Jill Smith") rather than a more formal address ("Dr. Smith") and encourage all other team members, including physicians, to do the same. This helps put everyone on an equal footing so they become more comfortable working together.

Although champions and opinion leaders can support patient safety efforts and improvement, responsibility for planning and implementing initiatives also rests with leadership. This means establishing teams, giving teams goals that reflect the hospital's mission and vision, training team members in the skills needed to achieve these goals, and allocating adequate resources for the project.

Setting Up Effective Teams

Before establishing a team for a specific initiative, it is a good idea to identify all the teams the hospital already has and exactly what they are working on. An existing team or committee may be able to include the new project in its charter, or a team that has been working on a similar project may no longer be needed—for example, the team has achieved the desired improvements and can now take on new or expanded responsibilities.

If no appropriate team currently exists, leaders will need to establish a project-dedicated, multidisciplinary team to work on the process or problem that has been identified as high risk. If a work committee already oversees this process, members from that committee may also be part of the patient safety team, but the patient safety team needs to be separate. Otherwise, the focus of the team will be fragmented between the day-to-day function of the process and improving performance to reduce risk. In setting up a team, leaders will need to address a number of questions, including the following:

- Who should be on the team?
- How will responsibilities be divided among team members?
- What are the team's goals?
- What training will team members need?
- What other resources will be needed for the initiative?

Composition and Responsibilities of the Team

The number of team members will depend on the complexity of the problem being addressed and the size of the hospital. A small community hospital team working on improving clinicians' compliance with hand hygiene procedures may include one representative each from the medical staff, nursing staff, and administration (materials manager). One or more of these team members may have additional roles such as quality improvement director or infection control specialist. In a large hospital that is part of a complex organization studying its communication among different settings, the team may be much larger. Representatives may be involved from nursing, medical staff, pharmacy, laboratory, therapy, medical records, and information technology from each facility, as well as leadership and quality professionals from the parent organization.

Individual roles and responsibilities within the team may be divided up in a number of different ways. The following are the most usual, although smaller teams may only have a sponsor, a leader, and team members.

Sponsor. The sponsor is a member of executive leadership and usually has ultimate responsibility for the area in which safety improvements will be made. The executive sponsor has several important responsibilities:

- Expressing the executive vision for improvement
- Providing senior management input and decision making, as necessary
- Serving as an information conduit between the team and executive leadership
- Ensuring that needed resources are available

- Offering ongoing support and encouragement
- Assisting with problem resolution as needed

A large hospital may have a quality oversight committee or other body that includes top leaders and fulfills this role.

Team Leader. This person is often the midlevel manager who has operational responsibilities for the area being addressed. He or she should be knowledgeable about operations and outcomes in this area. The team leader's responsibilities include the following:

- Gaining approval for and monitoring the budget for the project
- Coordinating team meetings, including scheduling, preparing agendas, assigning project work to be completed between meetings, and documenting team activities
- Creating and monitoring the implementation of the project work plan and time line
- Using and distributing the resources necessary to accomplish the team's mission
- Serving as an intermediary between the team and executive leadership
- Communicating regularly with the team sponsor about the team's work

Hospitalists are often good choices to lead teams because they are experts on their own facility. Unlike private practice physicians, who may spend an hour or two each day or several hours a few days a week at the hospital, hospitalists work there full-time and are knowledgeable about all the organizational systems and inpatient care. Their unique perspective allows them to see where processes may falter and how changes can best be integrated into daily care activities.[5]

Team Facilitator. The team's leader may also serve as its facilitator; however, if sufficient staff is available, it is helpful to have another individual perform this function. A facilitator may be an outside consultant or an in-house staff member who has received formal training in this area. He or she needs to provide an objective "outsider's" view, when team members who are closely involved in the process have trouble stepping back to determine whether they are on the right track.[6]

Although the roles of team leader and facilitator may be filled by a single person, carrying out both sets of responsibilities at the same time requires an exceptional ability to balance traditional management functions (such as staff supervision and financial control) with staff development through formal education and coaching. Although improvements can occur in a learning organization when one person performs the duties of both roles, that person may quickly become overburdened—especially if he or she is a physician who is already stretched too thin.

The facilitator has a number of responsibilities:

- Educating team members about the hospital's selected performance improvement (PI) method, improvement tools and techniques, and performance measurement and assessment
- Helping the team create and sustain an effective working dynamic
- Coaching the entire team and individual members in using performance measurement and improvement tools, collecting and analyzing performance data, generating and testing improvement ideas, and developing recommendations for hospitalwide changes
- Helping the team prepare for formal presentations to leaders
- Meeting with the team leader before and after meetings to analyze the effectiveness of the team process and plan process interventions, if necessary
- Providing support and encouragement

Team Members. As the backbone of the team, members complete the majority of the group's work. They are the physicians and staff who participate in—and whose daily tasks are affected by—the process being studied. Participants should come from all levels of these departments so the broadest perspective possible is represented. Because of their firsthand knowledge of how the process works in reality (as opposed to how it is supposed to work in policy), they can be considered subject matter experts. (See Sidebar 3-1, page 55, for other qualities to look for when assigning staff to teams.) The critical responsibilities of the team members include the following:

- Attending team meetings regularly
- Participating actively in all team meetings
- Completing between-meeting assignments

- Learning about and using PI tools and techniques
- Bringing issues, concerns, and problems to the attention of the team and team leader
- Supporting and promoting the project to peers and coworkers

Sidebar 3-1. *Team Member Characteristics*

In addition to expertise regarding the process involved, leaders may want to consider other criteria, such as the following, in selecting who will participate on a patient safety team. Note that these are also important characteristics of physician champions:

- Identified as an informal leader who is respected by peers
- Demonstrates interest in and knowledge of performance measurement/improvement methods and tools
- Displays creativity, good problem-solving skills, and the ability to think analytically
- Demonstrates commitment to continuous learning and improvement
- Demonstrates ability to work collaboratively with people in other disciplines
- Demonstrates an openness to new ideas

Sources: Scholtes P.R., Joiner B.L., Striebel B.J.: *The Team Handbook*, 3rd ed. Madison: Oriel, 2003, pp. 2–15; Skypek G.: Getting staff interested in performance measurement. *Joint Commission Benchmark* 5:11, Sep. 2003.

The responsibilities shown in the preceding lists are general and appropriate to any team. Specific responsibilities will vary according to the type of initiative being addressed and the individuals who participate. The roles different team members will play and how those roles will affect the success of the team must be considered up front. Even though actual assignments, deadlines, and so on will not be made until the team has been established, leaders can approximate the number of physicians and staff needed and how their knowledge and expertise can be used most effectively. It may be helpful to construct a matrix that sets out the anticipated members of a team and an overview of the tasks they will need to perform, as in Figure 3-1, page 56. This type of matrix can be used to plan for allocation of necessary personnel as well as to give time estimates to physicians who might be interested in participating (see Chapter 4).

Figure 3-1. *Team Member Responsibility Matrix*

Suppose that Wellness Hospital has identified a problem in turnaround times for laboratory and diagnostic test results performed for emergency department (ED) patients. Delays in treatment pose a significant risk to patient safety, and leaders have decided to form an improvement team to evaluate the process for problems and suggest ways to cut turnaround times. The initial responsibility matrix for this team (and other individuals who may be involved) might be similar to the one shown here.

Key:
P = Primary responsibility
S = Support (active involvement)
I = Keep informed
C = Consult or provide advice

	Collect and/or analyze data	Create flowchart of ED diagnostic / lab process	Review policies and procedures	Brainstorm ways to redesign process	Draft new policies and procedures	Educate staff about changes	Implement changes	Measure / compare performance to determine success
ED physician	S	P	P	P	P	P	P	S
ED nurse	S	P	P	P	P	P	P	S
Lab technician	S	P	P	P	P	P	P	S
Director of diagnostic services	S	P	P	P	P	P	P	S
Director of in-house transport services	S	P	P	S	S	P	P	S
Information management technician	P							P
PI staff member	P	S	S	S	S	S	S	P
ED director	S	C	C	C	C	P	P	S
Chief of medical staff	I				I	S	S	I

Source: Matrix adapted from Hartzler M., Henry J.E.: *Team Fitness: A How-To Manual for Building a Winning Work Team*. Milwaukee: ASQ Quality Press, 1994, p. 210.

An added benefit of planning out responsibilities is that it helps the team get up and running more quickly. If multidisciplinary collaboration is not yet an ongoing part of an organization, team members may have "turf" issues and expectations. If leaders already have an idea of what will be expected of each participant, the team leader/facilitator will have a basis from which to work in making specific assignments. This is not to say that the initial plan is carved in stone. Team members need to find the best way to work together toward their goals. This may necessitate making changes to leaders' original outlines, such as bringing in more people on an ad hoc-basis and shifting responsibilities among members.

Providing an Infrastructure

Chapter 2 examined how a learning environment and a culture of safety encourage collaboration and participation in initiatives. The foundation for successful teams is the organizational structure in which they function. Leaders need to invest in the team process as a whole: providing education and training, keeping lines of communication open, delegating authority to empower staff, supporting suggestions for change to fit with the hospital's mission and vision, and defining how success will be measured. If each of these elements is handled well, leaders build trust between themselves, physicians, and staff, which enhances the hospital's culture and encourages further participation in patient safety efforts.

To ensure that teams have been sufficiently empowered to make changes happen, it is a good idea to include at least some leaders of the organized medical staff in the participants. Because physicians tend to be goal oriented, they will be more likely to set ambitious goals and have the ability to achieve them.[2]

Developing Team Goals

For a team to function effectively, it needs a specific goal(s) toward which to work. A goal such as "to improve fire safety across the hospital" is too general to be of any use. The main goal of the project should be based on data that leaders, physicians, and staff have used to evaluate the hospital's programs. For example, if fire-drill logs show that staff in many areas do not know the correct procedures or take too long to evacuate the building, the team's goal might be "to ensure that all hospital personnel know and understand fire safety procedures and can demonstrate them in a timely fashion." This gives team members a starting point—they may attempt to find which areas have the poorest demonstration record; drill down to find the root cause(s) of a lack of understanding; and suggest changes to the scheduling and content of orientation, education, and in-services for all personnel.

In addition to being specific, patient safety project goals must align with the hospital's strategic goals, mission, and PI priorities. Leaders should consider the following questions when developing patient safety goals:

- Do data from ongoing PI activities show that there is a problem in this area?
- Will improvement of this process significantly reduce the risk of harm to patients?
- Have patient satisfaction surveys/patient complaints indicated that there is a problem in this area?
- Does improvement of this process coincide with the organizational mission, vision, and strategic goals?
- Is improvement in this area necessary to comply with government regulations, accreditation standards, or other mandated requirements?
- Will implementing improvements in this area require an increase in the operating budget?
- Will implementing improvements in this area improve efficiency and subsequently cut costs?
- Does this safety issue affect a large percentage of the patient population?
- Could an error in this process result in serious harm or death to a patient?

The more questions that are answered affirmatively, the more likely it is that the goal in question is appropriate to the hospital's needs.

Goals need to be realistic, given an organization's resources and needs. The need for improvement must be balanced against what is feasible. For example, Good Care Hospital may want to improve staffing effectiveness to reduce the number of patient falls. However, if the organization is experiencing shortages of physicians, nurses, pharmacists, and/or physical therapists, its goal must be less ambitious than it would be if full staff were available. The same holds true if a hospital is working on an initiative with other organizations. Each participating organization has its own strengths and weaknesses, so leaders must remember to keep their goals consistent with what is practical for their own facility.

> The reaction to the "To Err is Human" report was stupendous. Hospitals are trying to do better patient-safety management. . . . I recommend that all of the specialties do much of what the anesthesia world has done in patient safety. That includes establishing committees on patient safety, establishing research projects from the ground up on safety, setting up communication devices like our [Anesthesia Patient Safety Foundation] newsletter and establishing a huge interest in safety and culture. Hopefully, other specialties will move in that direction . . . .
>
> —Ellison C. Pierce, Jr., M.D., executive director and past president, Anesthesia Patient Safety Foundation. In Madell R.: Innovators in action. *HealthLeaders* 4(9):33–40, 2001.

Leaders shouldn't change goals too often. Many health care organizations set up their patient safety and improvement projects for one fiscal year; when that year is over, they choose new goals even if they don't have enough data to support these changes. Trying to move ahead to a higher performance level before the initial goal has been achieved is self-defeating for everyone. Physicians and staff become frustrated, and the hospital puts resources into projects that can't provide the desired outcomes because they haven't been given sufficient time.

Providing Training for Performance Improvement Team Members

Staff training is often a weak area in a hospital's patient safety and PI programs. To participate fully and effectively, individuals need to have a thorough understanding of patient safety issues, especially as they apply to the hospital. They also need some background in team dynamics and the PI process.

Skills for All Team Members

All participants need to have enough background in relevant patient safety issues to be able to make contributions to discussions and improvement efforts. Much of this background comes from experience, but certain topics may require additional education. For example, although team members may know that universal precautions help prevent the spread of infection, they may not know or follow the guidelines published by the Centers for Disease Control and Prevention (CDC). They also may not know that the Joint Commission's National Patient Safety Goals include adherence to the CDC guidelines on hand hygiene. The Web sites listed in Appendix A can provide a great deal of material on a wide range of patient safety topics.

According to Groff and Augello,[1] the following four skills are universally applicable to everyone working on any health care team:

- *Briefing.* This consists of having team members clarify the situation they're addressing and communicate effectively about what needs to be done.
- *Assertion.* All team members are empowered to speak up and express opinions.
- *Situational awareness.* Knowing how to stay focused on the issue at hand, as well as what indicates that discussion or work has gone off on a tangent, is important so the team's finite resources can be used effectively.
- *Debriefing.* A brief, specific discussion of what has gone well, what has not, what could be done differently, and what has been learned provides an opportunity for both individual and team education.

It is important to evaluate team members' knowledge of the hospital's PI process and plan education accordingly. The many sources of information on these and other techniques are beyond the scope of this book. However, leaders should plan to include training on PI techniques for each stage of the process. For example, methods such as flowcharting and brainstorming can be used to plan both the project as a whole and the actions to be taken to improve the process. Data collection is a large part of any improvement effort, so it is a good idea for team members to be aware of the various choices available when creating their tools. Data analysis is also an integral part of the process and requires at least a rudimentary understanding of statistical methods of interpretation. Table 3-1 below lists the various stages of the PI process and possible topics to address for each.

Skills for Team Leaders and Facilitators

Physicians or staff members who are chosen to lead/facilitate teams may need more specialized training than other team members to improve their leadership abilities. For example, people skills such as good interpersonal communication, listening, conflict resolution, and team building are necessary. Leaders and facilitators need to be able to train others on the team, which means they need to be well versed in various teaching methods. They may also need to learn technical skills such as using and interpreting statistics or organizing and planning projects.[2]

Table 3-1. *Tools and Techniques Used in Different Stages of Performance Improvement*

Initial Planning
- Brainstorming
- Cause-and-effect analysis
- Failure mode and effects analysis
- Flowcharting
- Multivoting
- Nominal group technique

Data Collection
- Check sheets/checklists
- Surveys (staff and patient)

Data Analysis
- Comparison charts
- Control charts
- Line graphs
- Pareto charts
- Run charts
- Scatter diagrams
- Stratum charts

Action Planning
- Brainstorming
- Cause-and-effect analysis
- Failure mode and effects analysis
- Flowcharting
- Multivoting
- Nominal group technique

> Improving patient safety incorporates two complementary approaches. The first . . . provides qualitative methods for anticipating errors, documenting critical incidents, and responding to them in a blame-free and structured manner. Using such qualitative methods, physicians can generate meaningful strategies for preventing similar occurrences in the future. Hospital-based physicians have an important role to play in promoting a culture of safety by championing incident-reporting initiatives and participating in multidisciplinary teams that analyze adverse events and promote change.
>
> The second approach involves applying the results of quantitative clinical research to reduce some of the common hazards of hospitalization. Hospitalists also have an important role to play in this arena because many of these safety targets and the associated clinical practices . . . are not on the radar screens of many hospital-based specialists.
>
> —Shojania K.G., Wald H., Gross R.: Understanding medical error and improving patient safety in the inpatient setting. *Med Clin N Am* 86:847–867, 2002.

Allocating Adequate Resources

All patient safety initiatives and improvement activities require leaders' investment and support in staff time, expert knowledge and help, technology, and money to achieve positive results. With concerns such as staffing shortages and decreasing reimbursement, leaders must often be creative in finding ways to come up with the resources a team needs. Finding resources may be challenging, but in the long run making a process better—and thus reducing or eliminating risks to patients—is cheaper than rework and litigation.

Staff Time

In addition to finding hours when physicians can take part, leaders need to give other hospital staff time to work on teams and projects. All leaders, middle managers, and direct-care staff must agree that participation in patient safety is a high-priority responsibility. Involvement in these projects should be included in all job descriptions and as a performance factor addressed at annual appraisals. Leaders need to encourage managers and staff to work together to find ways to ensure that staff participation in safety and improvement activities is routine without being disruptive to workers' care duties and other work processes.

Again, planning is key and requires input from front-line staff who will actually be involved. Only those who are part of the processes being studied will know the best ways to weave improvement activities into them. For example, if a hospital is measuring the effectiveness of a specific clinical practice guideline for preventing infection in joint replacement patients, attending physicians can complete brief data collection tools based on information they are simultaneously entering in the medical record. The tools can be included in all applicable records, then gathered and replaced at regular intervals. Or a hospital might try to gauge the number of emergency patients who require stat radiography. In this case, technicians who perform the x-rays could keep a tally on a simple daily check sheet as they work on each patient. It is important to make the tools used for measuring and improving safety as simple and easily available as possible.

Expert Knowledge and Help

Whatever types of initiatives are undertaken, a hospital needs to have someone who is knowledgeable about patient safety, PI, performance measurement, and the approach the hospital has chosen to take. This person should be available to leaders and staff to help with planning, coaching, and education. Some hospitals are able to dedicate one or more full-time employees to these functions, but many are forced to designate staff members who already have other responsibilities, whether in medical staff, nursing, human resources, or medical records.

If no staff members are available or there is no time to educate someone, leaders can try contacting community colleges, universities, or teaching hospitals in the area. Many of these institutions have or are developing curricula that include classes on total quality management and PI. Medical and nursing schools are offering more courses than ever in patient safety and proactively preventing errors. Students in all programs are often looking for opportunities to apply their knowledge and practice their skills in a real-world environment. Hospitals may be able to establish partnerships with academic institutions to create internships for these students and fill the human resource void.

Participating in national, state, and regional "quality projects" can also provide opportunities to interact with patient safety and PI experts. Volunteering to take part in pilot testing new performance measures, trying new clinical guidelines for a specific population, and so on can yield several benefits. Aside from the comparative information the hospital will receive on its own and other hospitals' performance, leaders and staff will have access to experienced professionals who can offer both formal and informal education and make recommendations about selecting and implementing patient safety and improvement initiatives.

If one or more staff members are available and willing to act as knowledge experts but require training to perform this function, leaders may consider membership in key professional organizations such as the National Association for Healthcare Quality (NAHQ) or the American Society for Quality (ASQ). Members have access to an entire network of people, projects, journals, books, and other resources dealing with PI. Association membership often results in learning partnerships among both individuals and health care organizations. Such partnerships provide opportunities for "no-cost" consultation, free or low-cost exchanges of staff education offerings, process benchmarking, and so on.

Resource people can also learn a great deal from key periodicals, including *Joint Commission Perspectives on Patient Safety™*, *Joint Commission Benchmark®*, *The Joint Commission Journal on Quality and Patient Safety™*, *Journal for Healthcare Quality*, *Journal for Quality and Participation*, *Quality Digest*, *Quality Progress*, and *Total Quality Management Review*. Regular review of these and similar publications can bring and keep staff up to date on patient safety issues, quality concepts, and PI processes. If one person does not have the time to read all the relevant material, the hospital can establish a "quality journal club" as part of its regularly scheduled staff meetings for all departments/disciplines. Each periodical is assigned to a different staff member, and readers summarize the pertinent information from their journal for others at the meeting. This strategy has the added value of engaging a wider number of staff in informal safety and improvement education.

The lessons that can be learned from other industries should not be overlooked. Both manufacturing and service organizations have been implementing worker safety, total quality management, and related approaches far longer than most of the health care field. Joining and participating in local business consortia can allow hospital staff to network with and learn from high-performing businesses within the community. Or leaders may be able to form a similar group with other health care organizations in the region, such as nursing homes, rehabilitation centers, behavioral health centers, and/or ambulatory clinics. Lessons learned in one setting can often be applied to others with a little creativity.

Finally, investigate how staff might participate in local, state, national, and international quality award programs. Volunteer reviewers and examiners for these awards are generally given substantial education about the intent, meaning, and assessment of award criteria—which generally translates into an intensive course in safety and PI. Although typically no fee is collected for training, participants may need to pay transportation and lodging costs. Reviewing award application forms, which are usually very detailed and specific, and thinking about their hospital's performance in relation to the award categories, gives physicians and staff a strong learning experience. They might even try completing a mock application for an award such as the John M. Eisenberg Patient Safety and Quality Award, cosponsored by the Joint Commission and the National Quality Forum, to gain a more in-depth understanding of their organization's infrastructure and how it actually operates in key areas.

Technology

Improving processes involves performance measurement, which includes collecting and analyzing complex clinical and nonclinical data for processes and outcomes. Software packages can help with many of the resulting data management issues, such as designing and using data collection tools, applying descriptive and analytical statistics, and visually demonstrating results. It is almost impossible for staff to measure, assess, and improve processes and outcomes without some sort of technological support, so leaders must realistically examine and address their hospital's technology needs.

If a large technology budget is available, leaders have a choice between many quality/PI or statistical process/quality-control software packages that are currently available. The sophistication, statistical capabilities, and graphic features of these products vary widely. Some are user-friendly, geared toward health care workers' "intuitive" appreciation for variations in performance, whereas others are more complex and require a greater understanding of statistical theory and application.

However, a hospital does not need the most cutting-edge bells and whistles to perform sound data analysis and interpretation. Staff may be able to adapt software they already have to collect, analyze, and present data. For example, if a facility uses one of the commonly available database programs, it may be able to insert appropriate formulas to have the software calculate run charts, control charts, and descriptive statistics. Even the most basic graphics packages can be used to create line graphs, bar graphs, Pareto charts, and other presentation forms. If the hospital is affiliated with a research or an academic institution, staff may have access to a comprehensive statistical package. This type of software can be used to calculate basic statistics, correlations, and control charts.

If there is simply no budget for technological support, a hospital can take the following steps to manage its data manually and effectively:

- Keep data collection tools simple
- Tally data counts often to avoid the necessity of working with huge stacks of data all at once
- Use calculators to determine rates, averages, and control limits
- Use a basic spreadsheet program such as Excel to draw simple data charts and graphs

Teams will still be able to use the information they gather to help focus on critical performance areas.

Financial Resources

All the resources already discussed require the outlay of financial resources to make them happen. The cost of staff time is usually the greatest measurement-related expense, followed by costs for training materials, technological resources, general supplies, and other expenses. If a hospital is addressing several initiatives at once or has decided to upgrade its current safety and improvement efforts, the costs for the year may be significant.

Leaders need to determine what the hospital can reasonably afford to invest in patient safety efforts. Another way of looking at the same question is asking whether the hospital can afford not to invest. The price of patient safety and PI cannot be viewed as simply another expense-driven cost center. Questions to keep in mind while making resource allocations and budget decisions include the following:

- Other than reducing risk to patients, what benefits will be gained from improving performance? How can effective PI reduce normal operating expenses?
- With the information obtained from improvement activities, can we prevent or minimize direct and indirect costs of errors (negative outcomes and near misses)?
- How much increased revenue will be realized from improvements to existing services?

Judgments about the importance of your safety and improvement activities cannot be made in a vacuum; they must take into account the impact of such activities on every area of the hospital.

Leaders have a limited amount of control over the use of the most valuable resources to any team—those who participate. Although hospital staff can be assigned, it is usually more difficult to pressure physicians into joining an initiative. Besides showing them the value of patient safety efforts (which has already been discussed), leaders must find ways to streamline both day-to-day and team activities to make them as time efficient as possible and persuade physicians that they will not become overburdened.

Case Study
Banner Desert Medical Center

When physicians are encouraged to find solutions to problems they've identified and that affect their patients, they become excellent advocates and team leaders/participants. Banner Desert Medical Center's Strategies to Eliminate the Progression of Severe Irreversible Sepsis (S.E.P.S.I.S.) Project was initiated by a physician and a nurse, and backed by medical staff. Located in Mesa, Arizona, Banner Desert is a Level 2 trauma center and is part of the largest not-for-profit secular health care system in Arizona, with 600 beds. It provides a diverse range of acute care services, including adult medical-surgical, critical care, and cardiovascular services. The Emergency Department (ED) sees more than 89,000 patients a year and the hospital has an average daily census of 470 plus patients. The intent of the S.E.P.S.I.S. Project was to reduce the overall mortality rate of critically ill septic patients and length of stay in the intensive care unit (ICU) by heightening the awareness of and using evidence-based treatments to combat the number one killer in the noncoronary ICUs.

Getting Started

Banner Desert became aware of the severity of the sepsis disease process through an evidence-based initiative carried out by the Surviving Sepsis Campaign (developed by the International Sepsis Forum, the Society of Critical Care Medicine, and the European Society of Intensive Care Medicine) and supported by the Institute for Healthcare Improvement. The hospital's mortality rates for sepsis patients had historically been high compared with rates of other patients, and sepsis was associated with a significant percentage of fatalities. The literature suggested earlier recognition and treatment—which includes early goal-directed therapy, appropriate antibiotics, administering drotrecogin alfa (activated), low-dose steroids for septic shock, intensive insulin control, and low tidal volume/high positive-end expiratory pressure in adult respiratory distress syndrome (ARDS)—could have a significant impact on the number one killer of critically ill patients in noncardiac ICUs. Banner Desert Medical Center developed the S.E.P.S.I.S. Project team to address this patient safety issue.

The project team, formed in 2004, was led by an intensivist and included representatives from the following areas:

- Critical Care Services (the director of nursing and an administrative assistant)
- Emergency Department (the department chair who is a physician, a senior clinical manager, a clinical nurse specialist, a service line coordinator, and medical associates)
- Intensive Care Unit (a senior clinical manager and clinical nurses)
- Quality Management
- Hospital coders
- House SWAT nursing (resource nurse for our hospital)
- Board-certified intensivists

The team distributed questionnaires to ED and ICU staff and physicians, including hospitalists, to determine whether this was a feasible improvement program to undertake. Many physicians felt the program would be a crucial way to combat sepsis and were eager in this process. More than 95% of the people who responded to the questions noted that sepsis identification and treatment are important, feasible, and achievable, but 30% of the respondents didn't feel like they would be able to identify septic patients and 60% weren't comfortable with the Surviving Sepsis Campaign guidelines.

Physicians were invited to participate and received meeting notices and e-mails regarding the S.E.P.S.I.S. Project meetings and educational components. They also received project updates through department meetings. These updates addressed three main issues: the problem of sepsis within the facility (high mortality, high cost, and high potential for improvement of care), new evidence-based treatments to manage it, and the collaboration of ED and ICU staff, as well as some hospitalists, to support and treat septic patients.

The project team then developed a new severe sepsis/septic shock protocol. The following key issues were addressed:

- Recognizing septic patients early
- Appropriate diagnostic workup for sepsis
- Accepting and implementing the protocol
- Evaluating the program to identify its effect on mortality reduction after implementation

The team's focus was on decreasing mortality, reducing medical errors, and improving consistency of care in critically ill septic patients using newer evidence-based practices. Tasks that could be delegated were completed by nursing and administrative staff from the ICU and ED.

Rolling Out a New Protocol

The S.E.P.S.I.S. Project team began educating staff about the new sepsis program with a teaser promotional advertisement that was posted in all areas of the hospital, including the ED and ICU. Critical Care Service, internal medicine, and emergency department meetings created time for discussions regarding severe sepsis and the significance of the protocol. Lectures were also presented to multiple nursing leadership and clinical leadership (shared leadership–Clinical Excellence Team, Quality Assurance, Banner Desert administration, and Practice Max–the ED shared leadership group), Medical Executive Committee, and several online educational lectures were given by the National Institute for Sepsis Education.

Banner Desert hosted a temporary intranet site that physicians, nurses, and all ED and ICU staff could use to learn more about sepsis. These intranet lectures addressed topics such as sepsis pathophysiology, early goal-directed therapy, and the Surviving Sepsis Campaign guidelines. CD-ROMs about managing and recognizing sepsis were made available for physicians and nurses. Staff was given a free S.E.P.S.I.S. T-shirt after completing the online education modules and accompanying quizzes.

Vendors sponsored dinner lectures to educate ED and ICU physicians and nurses about severe sepsis and currently available treatments. Two separate dinner lectures were held to allow more staff to attend. One speaker was an ED physician, and the second speaker was a Pulmonary/Critical Care Medicine physician. Both were actively involved in bringing the sepsis initiative to their facilities.

Immediately before the launch of the new sepsis protocol, Banner Desert hosted the First Annual Sepsis Symposium, which was coordinated by the S.E.P.S.I.S. Project team with major support from Eli Lilly and Company and Edwards Lifesciences, as well as other pharmaceutical and product companies. The symposium was promoted via e-mail and regular mail to hospital physicians, nurses, and administrators from the entire Phoenix area. Although physicians and nurses were the primary audience, attendees included coders, respiratory therapists, pharmacists, and administrators.

After the standardized sepsis protocol and educational processes were completed, the program was implemented. Changes were tested by determining how quickly septic patients were identified before and after protocol implementation and by measuring overall mortality rates for severe sepsis patients. Prior to the educational process, the number of severe sepsis or septic shock patients identified per quarter was 40 to 55 on average, with a baseline mortality rate of

33%. After the sepsis program was implemented, the average number of patients identified with severe sepsis/septic shock increased to 73 per quarter. The mortality had decreased to 25%, with the national average being 28.6%. The program expects even greater improvement as compliance with the sepsis protocol increases, with a goal of 95%.

In summary, the S.E.P.S.I.S. project helped raise the awareness of sepsis and engage physicians in improving patient safety and evidence-based sepsis care. This has been accomplished by identifying septic patients earlier and more efficiently, and by using sepsis-related, evidence-based practices to reduce unnecessary deaths. Hospitals in the Banner Health System are becoming more aware of the evidence-based projects being done in the ICU at Banner Desert Medical Center, and the project has helped clinicians maximize the delivery of patient-oriented, patient-safe sepsis care at Banner Desert as well as within the organization.

Sidebar 3-2. *Tips from Banner*

- Use resources available to you to help develop your patient safety initiative(s). Examples of these resources vary, including experienced facilities and clinicians involved in patient safety initiatives, standardized protocols, and data collection tools.
- Talk to others who have conducted a similar project.
- Have a unified vision for your initiative and note possible obstacles to its development and implementation.
- Make sure the administration is committed in both funding and actual support of the project.
- Work to obtain maximal support from clinicians and staff.
- Recruit "cheerleaders" from other disciplines.
- Think "big" but start "small." High goals are achievable if the path to them is broken down into manageable segments.
- Maximize time, energy, and resources by collaborating with other facilities.
- Don't give up. Remember, this is a patient-centered, evidence-based activity, and is not centered on the needs or demands of administration or physicians. It is for the patients.
- Share success stories with staff members. Show them they can make a difference.

References

1. Groff H., Augello T.: From theory to practice: An interview with Dr. Michael Leonard. *Forum* pp. 10–13, Jul. 2003.
2. Hellman R.: Improving Patient Safety in Diabetes Care in Hospital Settings—A Team Effort. Presented at *Moving from the Sidelines to the Frontlines of Patient Safety: Empowering the Medical Staff,* Chicago: Sep. 29–30, 2005.
3. Phillips, K.M.: *The Power of Health Care Teams: Strategies for Success.* Oakbrook Terrace, IL: Joint Commission on Accreditation of Healthcare Organizations, 1997.
4. Wexler D.: Give the birth dose! Providing all infants with hepatitis B vaccine at birth saves lives (letter), http://www.immunize.org/birthdose/letter.htm (accessed Oct. 9, 2001).
5. SHM Benchmarks Committee: Improving patient safety and quality of care. *The Hospitalist* 9 (Suppl 1):33–35, 2005.
6. Porter J.E.: The Benchmarking Effort for Networking Children's Hospitals (BENCHmark). *J Qual Improv* 21:395–406, Aug. 1995.

Chapter 4: *Facilitating Physician Participation in Patient Safety*

Physicians have been convinced of the need for improving patient safety. They have begun to believe in the possibility of improvement within day-to-day activities and have committed to helping in improvement efforts. A leader's work is done—right? If only it were that simple. Even with the best intentions, many clinicians simply do not have the time to attend all the meetings, read all the memos, and take part in all the steps necessary to make changes happen. Physicians already have numerous demands on their time, from private practice patients to hospital rounds to long term care resident visits. Some are also responsible for education, research, and/or administrative duties. An additional factor contributing to time constraints is the current shortage of physicians, especially in some specialties. A report commissioned by the Council of Graduate Medical Education, which advises Congress on physician work force issues, found that

> Communication failures are an extremely common cause of inadvertent patient harm. The complexity of medical care, coupled with the inherent limitations of human performance, make it critically important that clinicians have standardized communication tools, create an environment in which individuals can speak up and express concerns, and share common "critical language" to alert team members to unsafe situations.
>
> —Leonard M., Graham S., Bonacum D.: The human factor: The critical importance of effective teamwork and communication in providing safe care. *Qual Saf Health Care* 13(suppl 1):i85–i90, 2004.

the shortage could reach 85,000 physicians by 2020.[1] Medical areas with the most frequently reported shortages include anesthesiology, cardiology, gastroenterology, geriatrics, radiology, and general surgery.[2] Rural and inner-city primary care facilities are also facing shortages.

In researching the manufacturing and service industries, Frank Gryna found that several key causes contribute to work overload in all fields[3]:

- Insufficient resources to handle normal workload
- "Firefighting" problems
- A lack of control related to prioritizing, choosing work methods, and using resources
- Faulty work processes
- Unclear performance goals and responsibilities
- Missing/wrong/late input from internal and external suppliers
- Missing or poorly trained personnel
- Information overload
- Problems with information technology (hardware and software)

All these situations may be seen in hospitals and contribute to physicians feeling overwhelmed and unable to take on extra responsibilities. For example, problems in communication among caregivers can lead to delays in treatment, processes being followed incorrectly, and firefighting when errors occur. Poorly defined team goals and responsibilities mean that clinicians do not know how much time to allocate for patient safety initiatives; when more time than anticipated is needed, they may become overburdened or simply refuse to participate further.

To facilitate physician involvement and avoid work overload, leaders need to consider three main strategies: clearly defining responsibilities, improving communication on all levels, and streamlining processes to use time efficiently.

Defining the Scope of Physician Involvement

The ongoing day-to-day responsibilities physicians face combine with other factors to make the thought of joining a team singularly unappealing. These factors include the need for multitasking (answering pages, updating charts, taking phone calls, and so on), fatigue, stress (both professional and personal), and short-term memory (trying to remember all the information that comes to them each day).[4] Many clinicians have unrealistic expectations for themselves, believing they should be able to "do it all" and do it well. When this proves to be impossible, they become exhausted and frustrated, which ultimately leads to a higher risk for errors and less willingness to participate in patient safety initiatives.[5]

Before asking physicians to become involved with an improvement team, leaders must have a clear-cut idea of how much time will be needed. Time estimates are often unrealistic and do not include all the duties associated with a project. For example, knowing how many hour-long meetings are planned for the month is a good start, but preparatory work and review also take time. The following questions can be used to help consider the different activities in which a team member may be involved:

- Will the physician be operating in an advisory capacity, or will he or she be leading the team? (Team leaders require a far larger time commitment than other members.)
- How long will meetings last, and how often will they be held? Will the physician be required to attend all meetings or only strategic ones?
- What type of work will the physician be asked to do before coming to meetings (for example, researching best practices, getting opinions from medical staff)? How long should this preparation take?

- What other duties will the physician have (working with other members to create procedures, reviewing and commenting on other members' work, providing one-on-one education on changes to other clinicians, and so on)? How long might each task take?

It is important to remember that any perceived time estimate is often significantly less than the actual time required. To be realistic, it is a good idea to add another 20% to each estimate.[3] Although a higher number may put off some physicians, it is better to err on the side of caution. No one will complain if the actual time commitment is less than anticipated; however, a clinician who feels he or she has been misled and is forced to devote a great deal more time than originally predicted may be unwilling to continue with the project or refuse to take on team duties in the future. He or she may also be inclined to tell other medical staff members of the experience and discourage them from participating as well.

With a limited number of hours each day, a precious amount of time can be lost through poor communication among health care professionals—whether as part of a team effort or during normal care activities. Changes in this area can cut the time required for patient safety efforts and make care delivery run more smoothly.

Improving Communication

With the complexity of care today, it is essential that all caregivers—including physicians—have standardized communication tools and share a common language with other health care providers to avoid unsafe situations such as the following:

- Transferring incorrect or incomplete information from one provider to another
- Differing perceptions among caregivers regarding the same patient's needs
- Disrupting new processes and systems
- Introducing errors into existing processes

Communication failures have been identified as a root cause of 65% of all sentinel events reported to the Joint Commission, and hospitals have made communication issues (completeness, accuracy, timeliness, and clarity) a high priority for patient safety programs.

One of the main roadblocks to effective communication is the difference in communication styles among health care professionals. When calling a physician about a patient's condition, a nurse may provide a narrative description that gives an overall picture of the situation; the physician, however, prefers to hear a concise statement of a problem with a specific question or suggestion aimed at solving it.[4] He or she is not interested in the patient's entire history, only in those elements that are relevant to the current difficulty. To bridge this gap in communication styles, many hospitals are training staff to approach contacts with physicians in a different way, such as the Situational Briefing model, also known as SBAR (situation, background, assessment, recommendation), which is explained in more detail in Sidebar 4-1. Physicians are also being educated in how to ask for the information they want in a nonconfrontational

Sidebar 4-1. The Situational Briefing Model of Communication

Developed at Kaiser Permanente, the SBAR (situation, background, assessment, recommendation) technique uses a consistent approach to communication that allows for effective information sharing among physicians and other caregivers. Whenever hospital staff members contact a physician, they follow the process outlined here.

Situation: What is the situation you are calling about?

- Identify yourself, your unit, the patient, and the room number.
- Briefly state the problem, when it happened or started, and how severe it is.

Background: What background information is pertinent to the situation? Any of the following may be included:

- The admitting diagnosis and date of admission
- List of current medications, allergies, IV fluids, and labs
- Most recent vital signs
- Lab results, including the date and time the test was performed and the results of previous tests for comparison
- Other relevant clinical information
- Code status

Assessment: What is your assessment of the situation?

Recommendation: What do you recommend, or what do you want the physician to decide?

Source: Institute for Healthcare Improvement: *SBAR Technique for Communication: A Situational Briefing Model*. Institute for Healthcare Improvement. http://www.ihi.org (accessed Dec. 30, 2005).

way. Discussions that are clear and succinct reduce the amount of time required as well as the number of subsequent calls for clarification.

Another important consideration is communication between practitioners with different levels of experience in different areas. It is often difficult for health care professionals to realize that all caregivers are not operating from the same knowledge base. On patient safety teams, risk managers or quality improvement staff may quote statistics on nosocomial infection rates without putting the information into context for others on the team. Unless the numbers are presented along with their relevance to the hospital's population(s) and opportunities for improvement, it is probably just meaningless data to the rest of the group.

Similarly, in an academic hospital, an attending physician may not state problems and solutions clearly to residents, assuming they understand the reasons for each action taken. For instance, hand washing is a task that all caregivers are supposed to perform before and after touching a patient. An attending physician may wash his or her hands automatically without noting for residents what the proper procedure is, or explaining that the hospital has established guidelines for hand hygiene to try to reduce nosocomial infection rates, and that improving compliance with the guidelines is a current patient safety initiative. Or a teacher might diagnose a condition that seems obvious to him or her, and prescribe the appropriate medication, without clearly stating the problem and solution for the student. In either case, there is a risk that residents will not receive the information they need to provide high-quality care in the safest possible manner. Both physicians and staff need to be shown that completeness and clarity, as well as brevity, can save time and reduce risks.

It is important to note that striving for completeness can be a double-edged sword. Although everyone involved in an initiative needs to know what's going on and receive feedback on different aspects of the project, *everyone* does not need to get *all* the information about *everything*. Inundating physicians with e-mails, memos, and voice mails that do not directly concern them is one of the surest ways to cause overload. As with discussions about a patient, physicians want to know what the situation is and what needs to be resolved. Copying clinicians on every communiqué between every member of the team is unnecessary, time-consuming, and counterproductive. The following points should be considered when setting up lines of communication for patient safety initiatives:

- Decide at the beginning of the project who needs to be informed of what and make these decisions clear to team members. If participants feel they need more or less information, they will have the opportunity to say so.
- Use multiple but limited channels for communication. For example, if a process has been drafted by certain members of the team, it can be e-mailed or sent in memo form to others for review. If leaders or facilitators want to confirm meeting attendance beforehand, voice mail or e-mail can be used. In each case, it is an either/or decision; using both channels is overkill. It may help to let team members know up front what channels will be used for messages, because some people check e-mail far more frequently than voice mail or vice versa. Some prefer working with hard copy, whereas others like to edit online. Trying to accommodate members' preferences encourages their completion of tasks.
- Use team members' specific skills and knowledge to determine who needs to review what. For example, if a redesigned process is spread across three settings within the same hospital, representatives from each setting would be asked to comment on the issues that affect their area. This lessens the amount of work required of each member and concentrates his or her efforts where those efforts can produce the most benefit.
- As discussed for verbal communication, keep messages and instructions concise and clear.

Although communication is one of the most important processes to evaluate for time efficiency, others also contribute to overload if they do not run smoothly.

Streamlining Processes

The goal of many patient safety initiatives is to improve processes to reduce risk; however, the elements of the improvement process itself can prove cumbersome and in need of redesign as well. As discussed in Chapter 3, advance planning—including setting and prioritizing goals—is crucial to making any process work effectively. It is also necessary to make the steps in the process as time efficient as possible. Leaders need to examine how patient safety initiatives are conducted and how they can be structured to save physicians and staff valuable time.

For example, meeting attendance is often seen as the most onerous task of any project. Spending several hours discussing possible solutions to ambiguous problems can make even the most dedicated safety experts throw up their hands in frustration. Several time-management strategies can make meetings not only bearable but useful:

- *Scheduling.* Plan meeting times around physician and staff availability. Frequently, first thing in the morning is the best time to meet. Or choose scheduled breaks such as lunchtime. Because physicians typically have responsibilities outside the hospital, meeting by conference call may be the most practical solution. Many hospitals use their secure intranet site to post documents and presentations for use during conference calls.
- *Established times and agendas.* Send an agenda to all team members before the meeting. The agenda should include the start and end times, location (or phone number for a conference call), items to be covered, and who is responsible for presenting each item. Meetings should begin and end on time to be respectful of team members' other responsibilities and commitments.
- *Advance preparation.* To make the best use of meeting times, team members need to commit to being prepared for meetings. The team should set realistic goals for what needs to be accomplished at each meeting and then assign responsibilities as needed to meet those goals. If a team regularly fails to address most or all of the items on the agenda, the team leader or facilitator should evaluate the agenda for appropriateness.

This is only one part of the day-to-day routine that can be streamlined to lift a bit of the burden from physicians and staff who are participating in initiatives. Others may include communication problems, addressed earlier, and troubles associated with computers. Hospitals rely heavily on their computer systems, but clinicians and staff often have trouble using them—whether because of lengthy log-in procedures, a lack of compatibility from one area to another, or extended wait times for access to a terminal. If a problem arises getting information to those who need it, leaders need to work with their information technology department to resolve issues.

Persuading physicians to become involved in patient safety initiatives requires proving to them that the cause is worthwhile (discussed in Chapter 2), that improvement can be realized through a team effort (outlined in Chapter 3), and that participation in such efforts will not take up every spare moment they have. The best proof, of course, is the acknowledged success of an initiative that has already made a positive difference in patient outcomes. Being able to celebrate fewer near misses involving look-alike/sound-alike drugs, a decrease in fall rates among geriatric patients, or fewer surgical site infections can provide as much incentive as reward.

References

1. Hall, S.: Study predicts physician shortage. *Lansing State Journal Online Edition,* May 30, 2004. http://www.lsj.com/news/local/040530_docs_1b.html (accessed Dec. 30, 2005).
2. Cooper R.A., Stoflet S.J., Wartman S.A.: Perceptions of medical school deans and state medical society executives about physician supply. *JAMA* 290:2992–2995, 2003.
3. Gryna F.M.: *Work Overload! Redesigning Jobs to Minimize Stress and Burnout.* Milwaukee: ASQ Quality Press, 2004.
4. Groff H., Augello T.: From theory to practice: An interview with Dr. Michael Leonard. *Forum* pp. 10–13, Jul. 2003. http://www.rmf.harvard.edu/files/documents/Forum_V23N3_a5.pdf (accessed Dec. 30, 2005).
5. Bartlett E.E.: Always running behind? Try these time-management tips. *Med Econ* 76:83, Apr. 1999.

Appendix A: *Selected Resources*

Selected resources includes a list of Web sites, books, journal articles, and other publications associated with improving the safety and quality of care in health care. These selected resources represent a small portion of the organizations and literature that are available to leaders and should not be considered as all-inclusive of what is available.

Web Sites

Agency for Healthcare Research and Quality (http://www.ahrq.gov)
AHRQ sponsors, conducts, and disseminates research on improving the safety, quality, efficiency, and effectiveness of health care. The section titled "Quality and Patient Safety" provides links to a variety of tools, online journal articles, and free AHRQ publications that hospital leaders can use as resources for their own initiatives.

American Academy of Pediatrics (http://www.aap.org)
This Web site provides information on committee work, policies and guidelines, public policy and advocacy, and care delivery specifically related to pediatric patient safety.

American Academy of Orthopaedic Surgeons/American Association of Orthopaedic Surgeons (http://www.aaos.org)
Information about preventing medical errors related to surgery is presented here for health care providers and patients. Offerings for professionals include patient safety articles and presentations, sample standard order sets, and safety alerts. Most of the pages require an AAOS member password.

American College of Emergency Physicians (http://www.acep.org)
The Web site's search engine can link users to journal articles, publications that may be purchased, and other safety-related Web sites. A member account is required for use.

American College of Obstetricians and Gynecologists (http://www.acog.org)
This site's "Quality Improvement and Patient Safety" section includes ACOG Today articles on patient safety issues such as safe prescribing, new technology, regulatory requirements, and disclosing information about adverse events. There are also lists of tips for reducing risk in a variety of processes.

American College of Physician Executives (http://www.acpenet.org)
ACPE offers several courses on safety-related topics: techniques for

measuring and managing care, leadership skills for medical staff officers, and advanced quality management.

American College of Surgeons (http://www.facs.org)
This Web site has an online educational resource focusing on the morbidity and mortality conference that is a large component of quality improvement efforts involving surgeons. Pages are also devoted to ACS views on regulatory and legislative issues; preventing wrong-site, wrong-patient, wrong-procedure surgery; and patient safety principles for office-based surgery.

American Medical Association (http://www.ama-assn.org)
The AMA includes a wide range of material related to patient safety on its Web site. Topics include regulation and legislation, physician education, available conferences and publications, journal articles, and campaigns to improve safety and quality in patient care.

American Medical Directors Association (http://www.amda.com)
AMDA members can access a wide variety of online journal articles pertaining to federal, state, and professional issues regarding patient safety.

Anesthesia Patient Safety Foundation (http://www.apsf.org)
Established by the American Society for Anesthesiologists in 1985, the foundation's goal is to ensure that no patient is harmed by anesthesia. The Web site has a great deal of free material on current patient safety initiatives, grants, educational and clinical safety tools, technology, and news/events.

Centers for Disease Control and Prevention (http://www.cdc.gov)
A wide variety of safety-related information is available on this site, including National Center for Health Statistics error data; national programs and initiatives; government reports, policies, and regulations; infection control data; and workbooks on a host of safety topics.

Institute for Healthcare Improvement (http://www.ihi.org)
IHI brings together groups of health care organizations with a shared vision in its Breakthrough Series of projects; the focus is to produce

rapid system changes and improve outcomes while simultaneously lowering costs. The institute is also one of the national entities behind the 100,000 Lives Campaign that aims to prevent 100,000 avoidable deaths by June 2006 through improvement of patient care. Information about the campaign, enrollment forms, and intervention materials are all available on the Web site. Users can also sign up for safety-related programs and order IHI publications.

Institute for Safe Medication Practices (http://www.ismp.org)
The ISMP site includes educational resources for professionals, medication safety tools and resources, and industry news. Hospitals can report medication errors to the USP-ISMP Medication Errors Reporting Program and adverse drug reactions to the FDA's MedWatch. FDA Safety Alerts on medications and related devices are also published.

Joint Commission International Center for Patient Safety (http://www.jcipatientsafety.org)
Working with ministries of health and national patient safety organizations and experts, health care professional organizations, and patient/consumer groups, JCI focuses worldwide attention on patient safety solutions and best practices that can reduce risks to patients. The Web site's section for professionals and providers includes a section of tools and other resources, Web site links, journal articles, and products and services.

The Leapfrog Group (http://www.leapfroggroup.org)
The Leapfrog Group, which is made up of 170 companies and organizations that buy health care, works toward reducing the number of preventable medical errors and improving care quality. Hospitals may participate in the group's quality and safety survey; the resulting data are provided on the Web site to help consumers make informed choices about care. The site also has a set of National Quality Forum–endorsed safety practices ("Leaps") that are recommended for hospitals to improve patient safety.

National Patient Safety Foundation (http://www.npsf.org)
The NPSF site has numerous offerings for research, education and conferences, publications, and other resources related to patient safety. It

also sponsors various programs, such as Stand Up for Patient Safety for hospitals and Executive Sessions for health care leaders.

The National Quality Forum (http://www.qualityforum.org)
The NQF site provides information on developing and implementing a national strategy for health care quality measurement and reporting. The mission of the NQF is to improve American health care through endorsement of consensus-based national standards for measurement as well as public reporting of health care performance data that provide meaningful information about whether care is safe, timely, beneficial, patient-centered, equitable, and efficient.

Risk Management Foundation of the Harvard Medical Institutions (http://www.rmf.harvard.edu)
The foundation funds research grants to better understand patient safety issues, their etiology, and possible interventions. The section of the Web site that is open to the general public provides information about past and future grants; upcoming patient safety conferences; links to publications, articles, and handbooks; and a risk management glossary.

U.S. Food and Drug Administration (http://www.fda.gov)
In addition to its section on medical device safety, the FDA also offers an online video series about recalls, safety alerts, and patient concerns. MedWatch allows providers to report problems with products; view other reports related to products; and search for FDA safety information about drugs, biologics, and devices.

U.S. Pharmacopeia (http://www.usp.org)
The U.S. Pharmacopeia's MedMARx system, a national online database, aggregates hospital medication error data and disseminates it to participants. Organizations that contribute to the database (all reports are anonymous and use a standardized format) can access information about common types of errors and find examples of how other organizations have handled specific problems.

VA National Center for Patient Safety (http://www.patientsafety.gov)
As part of the Veterans Health Administration, NCPS promotes cultures

of safety to reduce and prevent avoidable harm to patients. Its Web site offers information on changing cultures; alerts and advisories for medical products and devices; hazard summaries; and tools for patient safety initiatives such as reducing falls, improving hand hygiene, and ensuring correct surgery.

Books, Journal Articles, and Other Publications

Aasland O.G., Forde R.: Impact of feeling responsible for adverse events on doctors' personal and professional lives: The importance of being open to criticism from colleagues. *Qual Saf Health Care* 14:13–17, 2005.

Blendon R.J., et al.: Views of practicing physicians and the public on medical errors. *N Engl J Med* 347:1933–1940, 2002.

Buerhaus P.I.: Lucian Leape on patient safety in U.S. hospitals. *Journal of Nursing Scholarship* Winter 36:366, Apr. 2004.

Casebeer L.L., et al.: Designing tailored Web-based instruction to improve practicing physicians' preventive practices. *J Med Internet Res* 5(3):e20, 2003. http://www.jmir.org/2003/3/e20 (accessed Nov. 25, 2005).

Cohen M.M., Eustis M.A., Gribbins R.E.: Changing the culture of patient safety: Leadership's role in health care quality improvement. *Joint Comm J Qual Safety* 29:329–335, Jul. 2003.

Joint Commission Resources: Error prevention: Physician education and collaboration are key. *Joint Commission: The Source* 1(2)7, Feb. 2003.

Gaba D.M.: Anesthesiology as a model for patient safety in health care. *BMJ* 320:785–788, 2000.

Goode L.D., et al.: When is "good enough"? The role and responsibility of physicians to improve patient safety. *Acad Med* 77:947–952, Oct. 2002.

Groff H., Augello T.: From theory to practice: An interview with Dr. Michael Leonard. *Forum* 10–13, Jul. 2003.

Gryna F.M.: *Work Overload! Redesigning Jobs to Minimize Stress and Burnout*. Milwaukee: ASQ Quality Press, 2004.

Haas J.S.: Physician discontent: A barometer of change and need for intervention. *J Gen Intern Med* 16:496–497, Jul. 2001.

Hellman R.: Improving Patient Safety in Diabetes Care in Hospital Settings—A Team Effort. Presented at *Moving from the Sidelines to the Frontlines of Patient Safety: Empowering the Medical Staff.* Chicago: Sep. 29–30, 2005.

Hershkowitz M.: Time stresses in the lives of physicians. *Med Health R I* 88:133–134, Apr. 2005.

Hoff T.J., Pohl H., Bartfield J.: Implementing safety cultures in medicine: What we learn by watching physicians. *Advances in Patient Safety: From Research to Implementation* (Volume I). Rockville, MD: Agency for Healthcare Research and Quality, pp.15–38.

Hosler F.W., Nadle P.A.: Physician-hospital partnerships: Incentive alignment through shared governance within a performance improvement structure. *J Qual Improvement* 26:59–73, Feb. 2000.

Landry M.D., Sibbald W.J.: Changing physician behavior: A review of patient safety in critical care medicine. *J Crit Care* 17:138–145, Feb. 2002.

Leonard M., Graham S., Bonacum D.: The human factor: The critical importance of effective teamwork and communication in providing safe care. *Qual Saf Health Care* 13 (suppl 1):i85–i90, 2004.

Palmer B.: *Making Change Work: Practical Tools for Overcoming Human Resistance to Change*. Milwaukee: ASQ Quality Press, 2004, p. 25.

Rosen A.B., et al.: Physicians' views of interventions to reduce medical errors: Does evidence of effectiveness matter? *Acad Med* 80:189–192, Feb. 2005.

Smith W.R.: Evidence for the effectiveness of techniques to change physician behavior. *Chest* 118 (2 suppl):8S–17S, 2000.

Sorokin R., Riggio J.M., Hwang C.: Attitudes about patient safety: A survey of physicians-in-training. *Am J Med Qual* 20:70–77, Feb. 2005.

Trowbridge R., Weingarten S.: Educational techniques used in changing provider behavior. In Shojania K.G., et al. (eds.): *Making Health Care Safer: A Critical Analysis of Patient Safety Practices.* Evidence Report/Technology Assessment No. 43 (prepared by the University of California at San Francisco–Stanford Evidence-based Practice Center under Contract No. 290-97-0013), AHRQ Publication No. 01-E058. Rockville, MD: Agency for Healthcare Research and Quality, 2001, pp. 601–606.

VanGeest J.B., Cummins D.S.: *An Educational Needs Assessment for Improving Patient Safety: Results of a National Study of Physicians and Nurses* [white paper]. National Patient Safety Foundation, 2003. http://www.npsf.org/download/EdNeedsAssess (accessed Oct. 19, 2005).

Waring, J.J.: Beyond blame: Cultural barriers to medical incident reporting. *Soc Sci Med* 60:1927–1935, 2005.

Weinberg R.M., Bhatt N.V., Vogenberg F.R.: Engaging physicians in cost savings initiatives: Eliminating medication cost bias in the selection of inpatient medications. *Physician Exec* pp. 12–18, Jan./Feb. 2005.

Appendix B: *2006 National Patient Safety Goals and the Universal Protocol for Preventing Wrong-Site, Wrong-Procedure, Wrong-Person Surgery™*

The purpose of the Joint Commission's National Patient Safety Goals is to promote specific improvements in patient safety. The goals highlight problematic areas in health care and describe evidence and expert-based solutions to these problems.

The Universal Protocol is intended to achieve the prevention of wrong-site, wrong-procedure, wrong-person surgery. It is based on the consensus of experts from the relevant clinical specialties and professional disciplines, and is endorsed by more than 40 professional medical associations and organizations.

2006 National Patient Safety Goals for Critical Access Hospitals and Hospitals

Goal 1: Improve the accuracy of patient identification.

Rationale: Wrong-patient errors occur in virtually all aspects of diagnosis and treatment. The intent for this goal is twofold: first, to reliably identify the individual as the person for whom the service or treatment is intended; second, to match the service or treatment to that individual.

Requirement 1A: ***Use at least two patient identifiers (neither to be the patient's room number) whenever administering medications or blood products, taking blood samples and other specimens for clinical testing, or providing any other treatments or procedures.***

Implementation expectations: The person-specific information is the "identifier," not the medium on which that information resides. Acceptable identifiers may be the individual's name, an assigned identification number, telephone number, photograph, or other person-specific identifier. Bar coding that includes two or more person-specific identifiers (not room number) will comply with this requirement.

Goal 2: Improve the effectiveness of communication among caregivers.

Rationale: Ineffective communication is the most frequently cited category of root causes of sentinel events. Effective communication, which is timely, accurate, complete, unambiguous, and understood by the recipient, reduces error and results in improved patient safety.

Requirement 2A: ***For verbal or telephone orders, or for telephonic reporting of critical test results, verify the complete order or test result by having the person receiving the order or test result "read back" the complete order or test result.***

Implementation expectations: Simply repeating the order or test result is not sufficient. Whenever possible, the receiver of the order should write down the complete order or test result or enter it into a computer, then read it back, and receive confirmation from the individual who gave the order or test result.

"Critical test results" are defined by the individual health care organization and will typically include "stat" tests, "panic value" reports, and other diagnostic test results that require urgent response.

Requirement 2B: ***Standardize a list of abbreviations, acronyms, and symbols that are not to be used throughout the organization.***

Implementation expectations: An official list of dangerous abbreviations, acronyms, and symbols has been approved by the Joint Commission and must be included on each organization's "Do Not Use" list. The official list is available at: http://www.jointcommission.org.

Additional items may be added to an organization's "Do Not Use" list at the organization's discretion.

The "Do Not Use" list applies to all orders and other medication-related documentation whether handwritten, entered as free text into a computer, or on pre-printed forms. It does not currently apply to computer-generated forms or displays. Trailing zeros may be used in non–medication-related documentation when a clear need exists to demonstrate a level of precision, such as for laboratory values, imaging study measurement of lesion sizes, or catheter and therapeutic tube sizes.

Requirement 2C: ***Measure and assess and, if appropriate, take action to improve the timeliness of reporting, and the timeliness of receipt by the responsible licensed caregiver, of critical test results and values.***

Implementation expectations: The organization will need to determine its current turnaround time for reporting.

The Joint Commission expects an organization to define the acceptable length of time:

- Between the ordering of critical tests and reporting the test results and values
- Between the availability of critical results/values and receipt by the responsible licensed caregiver. The organization then assesses these data, determines whether there is a need for improvement in the timeliness of reporting, and, if so, takes appropriate action to improve and measure the effectiveness of those actions.

Requirement 2D: ***Not applicable to hospitals.***

Requirement 2E: ***Implement a standardized approach to "hand off" communications, including an opportunity to ask and respond to questions.***

Rationale: The primary objective of a "hand-off" is to provide accurate information about a patient's care, treatment and services, current condition, and any recent or anticipated changes. The information communicated during a hand-off must be accurate to meet patient safety goals.

Health care has numerous types of patient hand-offs, including but not limited to nursing shift changes, physicians transferring complete responsibility for a patient, physicians transferring on-call responsibility, temporary responsibility for staff leaving the unit for a short time, anesthesiologist report to postanesthesia recovery room nurse, nursing and physician hand-off from the emergency department to inpatient units, different hospitals, nursing homes and home health care, and critical laboratory and radiology results sent to physician offices.

Implementation expectations: The following are attributes of effective "hand-off" communications:

- Hand-offs are interactive communications that offer the opportunity for questioning between the giver and receiver of patient/information.
- Hand-offs include up-to-date information regarding the patient's care, treatment and services, condition, and any recent or anticipated changes.
- Interruptions during hand-offs are limited to minimize the possibility that information fails to be conveyed or is forgotten. Hand-offs require a process for verifying the received information, including repeat-back or read-back, as appropriate.
- The receiver of the hand-off information has an opportunity to review relevant patient historical data, which may include previous care, treatment, and services.

Goal 3: Improve the safety of using medications.

Rationale: When medications are part of the patient treatment plan, appropriate management is critical to ensure patient safety. Developing standardized and redundant systems has been shown to decrease error and improve outcomes.

Requirement 3A: ***Not applicable to hospitals.***

Requirement 3B: ***Standardize and limit the number of drug concentrations available in the organization.***

Implementation expectations: When more than one concentration is necessary, the number of concentrations should be limited to the minimum required to meet patient care needs, such as may be the case in pediatrics or neonatal care, and those concentrations should be standardized. The Rule of Six, which results in individualized concentrations, does not meet the requirements of National Patient Safety Goal 3B. However, the Joint Commission will allow for extending the current exceptions process for using the Rule of Six through a transition to the expected use of standardized drug concentrations by all providers no later than December 31, 2008. Requests for exceptions will continue to be considered on an organization-by-organization basis and will require ongoing evidence of progress toward full implementation of the use of standardized drug concentrations.

The eligibility criteria for participating in the exceptions process during the transition period are as follows:

- The exception request applies only to the neonatal or pediatric acute care services provided by the organization.
- Emergent and nonemergent admixtures are prepared only by pharmacy staff in a sterile environment.
- Calculations respecting the drug solutions are validated during the preparation.
- The labeling of solution concentrations and drug per milliliter are clear to all caregivers, and the solution concentration (amount of drug per unit volume of solution) is clearly indicated on the label.
- If the Rule of Six is used in a pediatric setting, but standardized drug concentrations are used in other parts of the hospital, guidance aids are made available to caregivers who may not be familiar with one of these systems.
- If the organization has a neonatal intensive care unit, the pharmacy is open 24 hours a day to support the admixture service.
- Smart pumps are used. (A "smart pump" is a parenteral infusion pump equipped with IV medication error-prevention software

that alerts operators or interrupts the infusion process when a pump setting is programmed outside preconfigured limits. Smart pumps are designed to recognize prescription errors, dose misinterpretations, and keypad programming errors.)

Requirement 3C: ***Identify and, at a minimum, annually review a list of look-alike/sound-alike drugs used in the organization, and take action to prevent errors involving the interchange of these drugs.***

Implementation expectations: Multiple strategies are available to identify a list of look-alike/sound-alike drugs used in the organization. Three tables of look-alike/sound-alike drugs have been issued by the Joint Commission and are posted on the Joint Commission Web site (http://www.jointcommission.org). An organization must include on its own list a minimum of 10 look-alike/sound-alike drug combinations from these tables, in accordance with the instructions accompanying the tables. The tables include both generic and drug combination–specific prevention measures. Surveyors will expect to see several of the applicable prevention measures in place for each drug combination on the organization's list.

Requirement 3D: ***Label all medications, medication containers (for example, syringes, medicine cups, basins), or other solutions on and off the sterile field.***

Rationale: This risk reduction activity is consistent with safe medication practices and addresses a recognized risk point in safely administering medications in perioperative settings. Errors, sometimes tragic, have resulted from medications and other solutions removed from their original containers and placed into unlabeled containers. Medications or other solutions in unlabeled containers are unidentifiable. This unsafe practice neglects basic principles of medication management safety, yet has been routine in many organizations with respect to medications transferred to the sterile field.

Implementation expectations: Medications include any prescription medications; sample medications; herbal remedies; vitamins; nutriceuticals; over-the-counter drugs; vaccines; diagnostic and contrast agents used on or administered to persons to diagnose, treat, or prevent disease or other abnormal conditions; radioactive medications; respiratory therapy treatments; parenteral nutrition; blood derivatives;

intravenous solutions (plain, with electrolytes and/or drugs); and any product designated by the Food and Drug Administration (FDA) as a drug. Solutions include chemicals and reagents such as formaline, saline, sterile water, Lugol's solution, radiopaque dyes, glutaraldehyde, and chlorhexidine.

Medications and solutions both on and off the sterile field should be labeled, even if only one medication is being used. Labeling occurs when any medication or solution is transferred from the original packaging to another container. Labels include the name and strength of the medication or solution and the amount, if relevant and not apparent from the container. Labels can be developed by the facility or are commercially available; sterile labels can be purchased. All labels are verified both verbally and visually by two qualified individuals unless the same person prepares, labels, and administers the medication or solution. No more than one medication or solution is labeled at one time.

Any medications or solutions found unlabeled are immediately discarded. All original containers from medications or solutions remain available for reference in the perioperative area until the conclusion of the procedure. All labeled containers on the sterile field are discarded at the conclusion of the procedure.

At shift change or break relief, all medications and solutions both on and off the sterile field and their labels are reviewed by entering and exiting personnel.

Goal 4: Not applicable to hospitals.
Goal 5: Not applicable to hospitals.
Goal 6: Not applicable to hospitals.

Goal 7: Reduce the risk of health care–associated infections.

Rationale: Compliance with the Centers for Disease Control and Prevention (CDC) hand hygiene guidelines will reduce the transmission of infectious agents by staff to patients, thereby decreasing the incidence of health care–associated infections.

Requirement 7A: ***Comply with current CDC hand hygiene guidelines at http://www.cdc.gov/handhygiene.***

Implementation expectations: Staff should know what is expected of them regarding hand hygiene and should practice it consistently. Implementing all CDC guidelines with category IA, IB, or IC evidence is required (http://www.cdc.gov/handhygiene).

Requirement 7B: ***Manage as sentinel events all identified cases of unanticipated death or major permanent loss of function associated with a health care–associated infection.***

Implementation expectations: A significant percentage of patients/clients/residents who unexpectedly die or suffer major permanent loss of function have health care–associated infections. These unanticipated deaths and injuries meet the definition of a sentinel event and, therefore, are required to undergo a root cause analysis. The root cause analysis should attempt to answer the question "Why did the patient acquire an infection?" and, given the fact of the infection, "Why did the patient die or suffer permanent loss of function?"

GOAL 8: ACCURATELY AND COMPLETELY RECONCILE MEDICATIONS ACROSS THE CONTINUUM OF CARE.

Rationale: Patients are most at risk during transitions in care (hand-offs) across settings, services, providers, or levels of care. Developing, reconciling, and communicating an accurate medication list throughout the continuum of care is essential to reducing transition-related adverse drug events.

Requirement 8A: ***Implement a process for obtaining and documenting a complete list of the patient's current medications upon the patient's admission to the organization and with the involvement of the patient. This process includes a comparison of the medications the organization provides to those on the list.***

Implementation expectations: Organizations must implement a standardized method for creating an accurate list of medications at admission/entry and transfer. The list should include the full range of medications as defined in the accreditation manuals:

- Prescription medications
- Sample medications
- Vitamins
- Nutriceuticals
- Over-the-counter drugs

- Vaccines
- Diagnostic and contrast agents
- Radioactive medications
- Respiratory therapy–related medications
- Parenteral nutrition
- Blood derivatives
- Intravenous solutions (plain or with additives)
- Any product designated by the FDA as a drug

Developing a medication reconciliation form to be used as a template for gathering information about current medications is one method that can be used to standardize care and prevent errors.

Requirement 8B: ***A complete list of the patient's medications is communicated to the next provider of service when a patient is referred or transferred to another setting, service, practitioner, or level of care within or outside the organization.***

Implementation expectations: The patient's accurate medication reconciliation list (complete with medications prescribed by the first provider of service) is communicated to the next provider of service, whether it be within or outside the organization. Thereafter, the next provider of service should check over the medication reconciliation list again to make sure it is accurate and in concert with any new medications to be ordered/prescribed.

At a minimum, reconciliation must occur any time the organization requires that orders be rewritten and any time the patient changes service, setting, provider, or level of care and new medication orders are written. For transitions not involving new medications or rewriting of orders, the organization should determine whether reconciliation must occur.

Goal 9: Reduce the risk of patient harm resulting from falls.

Rationale: Falls account for a significant portion of injuries in hospitalized patients, long term care residents, and home care recipients. In the context of the population it serves, the services it provides, and its environment of care, the organization should assess its patients' risk for falls and take action to reduce the risk of falling and to reduce the risk of injury, should a fall occur.

Requirement 9B: ***Implement a fall reduction program and evaluate the effectiveness of the program.***

Implementation expectations: As appropriate to the population served, the services provided, and the environment of care, a fall reduction program may include risk assessment and periodic reassessment of individual patients or of the environment of care. The program should include risk reduction strategies, in-services, and involving patients/families in education and environment of care redesign. The program should also include developing and implementing transfer protocols (for example, bed-to-chair), when relevant.

The Universal Protocol

Wrong-site, wrong-procedure, wrong-person surgery can be prevented. The Universal Protocol is intended to achieve that goal. It is based on the consensus of experts from the relevant clinical specialties and professional disciplines, and is endorsed by more than 40 professional medical associations and organizations.

In developing this protocol, experts reached consensus on the following principles:

- Wrong-site, wrong-procedure, wrong-person surgery can and must be prevented.
- A robust approach—using multiple, complementary strategies—is necessary to achieve the goal of eliminating wrong-site, wrong-procedure, wrong-person surgery.
- Active involvement and effective communication among all members of the surgical team is important for success.
- To the extent possible, the patient (or legally designated representative) should be involved in the process.
- Consistently implementing a standardized approach using a universal consensus-based protocol will be most effective.
- The protocol should be flexible enough to allow for implementation with appropriate adaptation when required to meet specific patient needs.
- A requirement for site marking should focus on cases involving right/left distinction, multiple structures (fingers, toes), or various levels (spine).
- The universal protocol should be applicable or adaptable to all operative and other invasive procedures that expose patients to

harm, including procedures done in settings other than the operating room.

In concert with these principles, the following steps, taken together, constitute the Universal Protocol for eliminating wrong-site, wrong-procedure, wrong-person surgery:

- Preoperative verification process
  - *Purpose:* To ensure that all the relevant documents and studies are available prior to the start of the procedure, they have been reviewed, and they are consistent with each other and with the patient's expectations and with the team's understanding of the intended patient, procedure, site and, as applicable, any implants. Missing information or discrepancies must be addressed before starting the procedure.
  - *Process:* An ongoing process of information gathering and verification, beginning with the determination to do the procedure, continuing through all settings and interventions involved in the preoperative preparation of the patient, up to and including the "time-out" just before the start of the procedure.
- Marking the operative site
  - *Purpose:* To identify unambiguously the intended site of incision or insertion.
  - *Process:* For procedures involving right/left distinction, multiple structures (such as fingers and toes), or multiple levels (as in spinal procedures), the intended site must be marked such that the mark will be visible after the patient has been prepped and draped.
- "Time-out" immediately before starting the procedure
  - *Purpose:* To conduct a final verification of the correct patient, procedure, site and, as applicable, implants.
  - *Process:* Active communication among all members of the surgical/procedure team, consistently initiated by a designated member of the team, conducted in a "fail-safe" mode; that is, the procedure is not started until any questions or concerns are resolved.

UP 1

The organization fulfills the expectations set forth in the Universal Protocol for Preventing Wrong Site, Wrong Procedure, Wrong Person Surgery™ and associated implementation guidelines.

Requirement 1A

Conduct a preoperative verification process as described in the Universal Protocol.

Requirement 1B

Mark the operative site as described in the Universal Protocol.

Requirement 1C

Conduct a "time-out" immediately before starting the procedure, as described in the Universal Protocol.

Implementation Expectations for the Universal Protocol

These guidelines provide detailed implementation requirements, exemptions, and adaptations for special situations.

Preoperative Verification Process

Verification of the correct person, procedure, and site should occur as follows (as applicable):

- At the time the surgery/procedure is scheduled
- At the time of admission or entry into the facility
- Any time the responsibility for care of the patient is transferred to another caregiver
- With the patient involved, awake and aware, if possible
- Before the patient leaves the preoperative area or enters the procedure/surgical room

A preoperative verification checklist may be helpful to ensure availability and review of the following, prior to the start of the procedure:

- Relevant documentation (for example, H&P, consent)
- Relevant images, properly labeled and displayed
- Any required implants and special equipment

Marking the Operative Site

- Make the mark at or near the incision site. Do NOT mark any nonoperative site(s) unless necessary for some other aspect of care.
- The mark must be unambiguous (for example, use initials or "YES" or a line representing the proposed incision; consider that "X" may be ambiguous).
- The mark must be positioned to be visible after the patient is prepped and draped.
- The mark must be made using a marker that is sufficiently permanent to remain visible after completion of the skin prep. Adhesive site markers should not be used as the sole means of marking the site.
- The method of marking and type of mark should be consistent throughout the organization.
- At a minimum, mark all cases involving laterality, multiple structures (fingers, toes, lesions), or multiple levels (spine). ***Note:*** In addition to preoperative skin marking of the general spinal region, special intraoperative radiographic techniques are used for marking the exact vertebral level.
- The person performing the procedure should do the site marking.
- Marking must take place with the patient involved, awake, and aware, if possible.
- Final verification of the site mark must take place during the "time-out."
- A defined procedure must be in place for patients who refuse site marking.
- Exemptions:
  - — Single organ cases (for example, cesarean section, cardiac surgery).
  - — Interventional cases for which the catheter/instrument insertion site is not predetermined (for example, cardiac catheterization).
  - — Teeth—BUT indicate operative tooth name(s) on documentation OR mark the operative tooth (teeth) on the dental radiographs or dental diagram.
  - — Premature infants, for whom the mark may cause a permanent tattoo.

"Time-Out" Immediately Before Starting the Procedure

Must be conducted in the location where the procedure will be done, just before starting the procedure. It must involve the entire operative team, use active communication, be briefly documented, such as in a checklist (the organization should determine the type and amount of documentation) and must, at the least, include the following:

- Correct patient identity
- Correct side and site
- Agreement on the procedure to be done
- Correct patient position
- Availability of correct implants and any special equipment or special requirements

The organization should have processes and systems in place for reconciling differences in staff responses during the "time-out."

Procedures for Non–OR Settings, Including Bedside Procedures

- Site marking must be done for any procedure that involves laterality, multiple structures or levels (even if the procedure takes place outside an OR).
- Verification, site marking, and "time-out" procedures should be as consistent as possible throughout the organization, including the OR and other locations where invasive procedures are done.
- Exception: Cases in which the individual doing the procedure is in continuous attendance with the patient from the time of decision to do the procedure and consent from the patient through to the conduct of the procedure may be exempted from the site marking requirement. The requirement for a "time-out" final verification still applies.

Index

A

Academic detailing technique, 36–37
Academic hospitals, 28–30
Adverse events
  in communication failures, 76
  complacency on, 15, 24, 32
  contributing factors in, 3–5
  death rate in, 2, 6, 12
    in sepsis, 68–71
  denial of, 15, 24
  hierarchical issues in, 15, 24–25
  incidence and outcome of, 1–2
  and learning opportunities in near misses, 27–28
  physician attitudes toward, 10–15
  proactive approach to, 26–27
  punitive reactions to, 2, 15, 25
  reporting of. *See* Reporting of adverse events
  root causes of, 10, 11, 27, 76
  Swiss Cheese Model of, 3–5
  tolerance of, 15, 24
Agency for Healthcare Research and Quality, 84
  on priority areas for patient safety improvements, 7
  survey on patient safety culture, 28
  Web site resources of, 40, 84
American Academy of Orthopedic Surgeons, 84
American Academy of Pediatrics, 84
American Association of Orthopedic Surgeons, 84
American College of Emergency Physicians, 84
American College of Obstetricians and Gynecologists, 84
American College of Physician Executives, 84–85
American College of Physicians, 40
American College of Surgeons, 85
American Medical Association, 8, 85
American Medical Directors Association, 85
American Society for Quality, 64
Anesthesia Patient Safety Foundation, 85
Aron, D. C., 50
Attitudes toward patient safety, 10–15
  educational strategies for change in, 23–44
Audit process in educational interventions, 37, 39
Augello, T., 60
Autonomy issues in team approach, 13, 48

B

Banner Desert Medical Center case study, 68–71
Barriers to patient safety interventions
  financial issues in, 14, 66–67
  physician attitudes in, 10–15
    educational strategies for change in, 23–44
  time constraints in. *See* Time constraints affecting patient safety interventions

Best practices
in learning culture, 28
views of local opinion leaders on, 37–38
Bonacum, D., 74
Briefing technique
in situational briefing model of communication, 77
in teams, 60
Brooke Army Medical Center case study, 42–44

C

Case studies
on Banner Desert Medical Center, 68–71
on Brooke Army Medical Center, 42–44
on University of Michigan Health System, 17–19
Catheter-related infections, 7, 8–9
Centers for Disease Control and Prevention, 60, 85
Centers for Medicare & Medicaid Services, 6
Change process
barriers to, 10–15
complacency affecting, 15, 24, 32
denial of need for, 15, 24
educational strategies in, 23–44
facilitation of physician participation in, 73–81
motivation affecting, 15, 24, 48
opinion leaders in, 37–38, 39, 49–51
potential benefits in, 32–34, 48–49
skepticism on need for, 12–13, 48, 49
team approach to, 47–71
Chief medical officer as leader in patient safety initiatives, 31
Classen, David C., 27
Cohen, Max M., 15
Collaboration
of leaders in patient safety initiatives, 31
in multidisciplinary team, 57
in teaching hospitals, 29
Communication, 74, 76–79
completeness and clarity of, 78
national patient safety goals on, 92–94
in sentinel events, 76
in situational briefing model, 77
in teams, 60
potential overload in, 78–79
Complacency about errors and adverse events, 15, 24, 32
Computerized physician order entry, 32–35
Cost issues. *See* Financial issues
Covey, Stephen R., 26
Crossing the Quality Chasm: A New Health System for the 21st Century, 6
Culture, organizational
barriers to patient safety interventions in, 10–15
complacency on errors and adverse events in, 15, 24, 32
denial of errors and adverse events in, 15, 24
educational strategies for change in, 23–44
hierarchical issues in, 15, 24–25
physician champions and opinion leaders affecting, 51

in teaching hospitals, 28–29
survey assessment of, 28, 33
teamwork in, 47–71
tolerance of errors and adverse events in, 15, 24

D

Data collection and analysis
skills of team members on, 60–61
technology required for, 65–66
time required for, 63
Death rate in adverse events, 2, 6, 12
in sepsis, 68–71
Debriefing meetings, 37, 60
Defense Department patient safety program, 44
Denial of errors and adverse events, 15, 24
Device-related infections, 7, 8–9
in University of Michigan Health System safety initiative, 17
Distance-learning program in Brooke Army Medical Center, 42–44
Drug errors and adverse events, 8
academic detailing education technique on, 36–37
computerized physician order entry system in prevention of, 32–35
Education Compass model on, 29–30
national patient safety goals on, 94–97, 98–99
in University of Michigan Health System safety initiative, 17

E

Early adopters, 49
Education and training, 11–12, 23–44
academic detailing technique in, 36–37
in academic hospitals, 28–30
affecting completeness and clarity of communication, 78
audit and feedback processes in, 37, 39
on benefits of patient safety improvements, 32–34
books, journals, and publication resources in, 64, 88–90
case study on Brooke Army Medical Center, 42–44
collaboration of leaders in, 31
debriefing meetings in, 37, 60
in Education Compass model, 29–30
effectiveness of, 34–39
opinion leaders in, 37–38, 39
on performance improvement techniques, 60–61
proactive approach in, 39
reminder systems in, 37, 39
on sepsis protocol, 70
simulation of preferred practices in, 37
of team members, 55, 59–61, 63–65
Web site resources in, 38, 40–41, 60, 84–88
of Defense Department, 44
Education Compass model, 29–30
Environmental factors in adverse events, 4, 5
Eustis, Mark A., 15
Expert knowledge, 63–65

F
Facilitator of team, 53–54
  skills of, 61
Fall risk reduction
  national patient safety goals on, 99–100
  in University of Michigan Health System, 17
Feedback process in educational interventions, 37, 39
Financial issues
  in Education Compass model, 29, 30
  in team activities, 67
  in time constraints on physicians, 14
Fire safety procedures, 57–58
Flanders, Scott, 17
Food and Drug Administration, 87

G
Graham, S., 74
Gribbins, Ronald E., 15
Groff, H., 60
Gross, Richard, 10, 62
Gryna, Frank, 74

H
Headrick, Linda A., 29, 50
Health Alliance of Central New York, 31
Hellman, Richard, 38
Hepatitis B virus vaccination in newborns, 50
Hernia surgery, 2–3
Hierarchical issues in organization culture, 15, 24–25
  physician champions and opinion leaders affecting, 51
  in teaching hospitals, 28–29
Hoff, T. J., 28
Hospital Compare, 6
Hospital Quality Alliance, 6
Hospitalists as Emerging Leaders in Patient Safety initiative at University of Michigan Health System, 17–19

I
Identification of patients, national safety goals on, 92
Infection control, 8–9
  in Banner Desert Medical Center, 68–71
  national patient safety goals on, 97–98
  opportunities for improvements in, 7
  physician champions in, 50
  postoperative, 6, 7, 9
  universal precautions in, 60
  in University of Michigan Health System, 17
Institute for Healthcare Improvement, 8–9, 85–86
Institute for Safe Medication Practices, 86
Institute of Medicine, 5–6, 12, 59

J
Joint Commission
  National Patient Safety Goals, 6, 60, 91–100
  quality of care data, 6
  Universal Protocol, 6, 91, 100–104
Joint Commission International Center for Patient Safety, 40, 86

K

Ketring, Susan Penn, 2
Kilbridge, Peter M., 27

L

Leadership
 collaboration in patient safety initiatives, 31
 as contributing factor in adverse events, 5
 facilitating physician participation in patient safety, 73–81
 in learning organizations, 25–26
 opinion leaders in
  in educational strategies, 37–38, 39
  in team approach, 49–51
 principle-centered, 26
 team leaders in, 53
  in goal development, 58–59
  in resource allocation, 62–67
  skills of, 61
Leape, Lucian L., 9
Leapfrog Group, 6, 86
Learning organizations, 25–39
 best practices in, 28
 proactive approach to patient safety in, 26–27
 value of near misses in, 27–28
Leonard, M., 74
Lowenhaupt, Manuel, 48

M

Making Health Care Safer: A Critical Analysis of Patient Safety Practice, 7
Making Strides in Safety campaign of AMA, 8
Medication errors. *See* Drug errors and adverse events
Medscape patient safety education resources, 40
Missouri Baptist Medical Center, 31
Mortality rate in adverse events, 2, 6, 12
 in sepsis, 68–71
Motivation for change, 15, 24, 48
Multidisciplinary teams. *See* Teams
Myocardial infarction, patient safety and quality of care in, 6, 8, 9

N

National Association for Healthcare Quality, 64
National Patient Safety Foundation, 15, 24, 35, 86–87
 Web site resources of, 41, 86–87
National Patient Safety Goals, 6, 60, 91–100
 in Brooke Army Medical Center case study, 42
National Quality Forum, 87
Nelson, John C., 8

O

100,000 Lives campaign of the Institute for Healthcare Improvement, 8–9
One-on-one education, 36–37
Opinion leaders
 in educational strategies, 37–38, 39
 in team approach, 49–51

P

Patient factors in adverse events, 5
Patient identification, national safety goals on, 92

Performance improvement
stages of, 61
streamlining of processes in, 63, 79–81
training of team members on techniques in, 60–61, 63–65
Physicians
attitudes towards patient safety, 10–15
educational strategies for change in, 23–44
facilitating participation in patient safety, 73–81
as opinion leaders
in educational strategies, 37–38, 39
in team approach, 49–51
shortage in number of, 73–74
as team members, 47–71. *See also* Teams, physician involvement in
Pierce, Ellison C., Jr., 59
Pneumonia, 6, 17
ventilator-associated, 7, 9
Preferred practices, simulation of, 37
Preston, Paul G., 24
Principle-centered leadership, 26
Proactive approach to patient safety, 26–27
educational strategies in, 39
Process factors in adverse events, 3, 4, 5
Punitive reactions to adverse events, 2, 15, 25

Q

Quality of care, Web site information on, 6
Questionnaire on organizational safety culture, 28, 33

R

Reason, James, 3
Reminder systems on care guidelines, 37, 39
Reporting of adverse events
in learning organizations, 27–28
motivation for, 15, 24
skepticism on data in, 12–13
in teaching hospitals, 28–29
Resource allocation to team activities, 62–67
Risk Management Foundation of the Harvard Medical Institutions, 87
Root causes of sentinel events, 10, 11, 27
in communication failures, 76

S

Senge, Peter M., 25–26
Sentinel events. *See also* Adverse events
in communication failures, 76
incidence of, 1–2
root causes of, 10, 11, 27, 76
Sepsis management in Banner Desert Medical Center, 68–71
Shojania, Kaveh G., 10, 62
Simulation of preferred practices, 37
Situational awareness of team members, 60
Situational briefing model of communication, 77
Skepticism of physicians on patient safety interventions, 12–13
in team approach, 48, 49
Society of Academic Emergency Medicine, 41
Software packages for data collection and analysis, 65–66

Sponsor of team, 52–53
Status quo, satisfaction with, 15, 24, 32
Strategies to Eliminate the Progression of Severe Irreversible Sepsis (S.E.P.S.I.S.) project, 68–71
Surgery
infection control in, 6, 7, 9
multiple sources of adverse outcomes in, 2–3
wrong-site, wrong-procedure, wrong-patient, 6
Universal Protocol in prevention of, 6, 91, 100–104
Survey on organizational safety culture, 28, 33
Swiss Cheese Model, 3–5
Systems approach to patient safety, 2–5

T

Teaching hospitals, 28–30
Teams
communication in, 60
potential overload in, 78–79
composition of, 51–57
empowerment of, 57, 60
establishment of, 51–57
existing, identification of, 51
facilitator of, 53–54
skills of, 61
goals of, 57–59
questions considered in development of, 58
leaders of, 53
in goal development, 58–59
in resource allocation, 62–67
skills of, 61
meeting attendance in, 80
organizational structure of, 57
physician involvement in, 47–71
autonomy issues in, 13, 48
facilitation of, 73–81
hierarchical issues in, 51
opinion leaders or physician champions affecting, 49–51
potential benefits of, 48–49, 67
skepticism about, 48, 49
time required for, 73–76, 80
resources required, 62–67
expert knowledge and training, 63–65
financial, 67
technology, 65–66
time, 62–63, 73–76, 80
responsibilities of members, 51–57
defining scope of, 75–76
matrix on, 55, 56
sponsor of, 52–53
training and skills of members in, 55, 59–61, 63–65
Technology
in computerized physician order entry system, 32–35
as contributing factor in adverse events, 4, 5
team requirements for, 65–66
Time constraints affecting patient safety interventions, 14, 48, 62–63, 73–76
in communication overload, 78–79
in financial cutbacks, 14
in team meetings, 80

To Err is Human: Building a Safety Health System, 6, 59
Tolerance of errors and adverse events in organizational culture, 15, 24
Training and education, 11–12, 23–44. *See also* Education and training

U

Universal precautions for infection control, 60
Universal Protocol in surgery, 6, 91, 100–104
University of Michigan Health System case study, 17–19
U.S. Pharmacopeia, 87

V

VA National Center for Patient Safety, 41, 87–88
Ventilator-associated pneumonia, 7, 9
Video-based distance-learning in Brooke Army Medical Center, 42–44

W

Wald, Heidi, 10, 62
Web sites
  as educational resource on patient safety, 38, 40–41, 60, 84–88
    of Defense Department, 44
  on patient safety culture survey, 28
  on quality of care, 6
WebMD, 40
Wenneker, Mark B., 31
West Virginia University Pharmacy School, 36
White, James P., 2
Wrong-site, wrong-procedure, wrong-patient surgery, 6
  Universal Protocol on prevention of, 6, 91, 100–104